New World Choreographies

Series Editors
Rachel Fensham
School of Culture and Communication
University of Melbourne
Parkville, Australia

Peter M. Boenisch
Royal Central School of Speech and Drama
London, UK

This series presents advanced yet accessible studies of a rich field of new choreographic work which is embedded in the global, transnational and intermedial context. It introduces artists, companies and scholars who contribute to the conceptual and technological rethinking of what constitutes movement, blurring old boundaries between dance, theatre and performance. The series considers new aesthetics and new contexts of production and presentation, and discusses the multi-sensory, collaborative and transformative potential of these new world choreographies.

More information about this series at
http://www.palgrave.com/gp/series/14729

Lise Uytterhoeven

Sidi Larbi Cherkaoui

Dramaturgy and Engaged Spectatorship

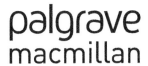

Lise Uytterhoeven
London Studio Centre
London, UK

New World Choreographies
ISBN 978-3-030-27815-1   ISBN 978-3-030-27816-8   (eBook)
https://doi.org/10.1007/978-3-030-27816-8

Cover credit: Koen Broos

This Palgrave Macmillan imprint is published by the registered company Springer Nature Switzerland AG
The registered company address is: Gewerbestrasse 11, 6330 Cham, Switzerland

To Mia

Series Editors' Preface

Choreography in the global context of the twenty-first century involves performance practices that are often fluid, mediated, interdisciplinary, collaborative and interactive. Choreographic projects and choreographic thinking circulate rapidly within the transnational flows of contemporary performance, prompting new aesthetics and stretching the disciplinary boundaries of established 'dance studies'. Crossing the borders of arts disciplines, histories and cultures, these 'new world choreographies' utilise dance techniques and methods to new critical ends in the body's interaction with the senses, the adoption of technology, the response to history as well as present-day conditions of political and social transformation, or in its constitution of spectator communities.

As a result, well-rehearsed approaches to understanding choreography through dance lineages, canonical structures or as the product of individual artists give way to new modes of production and representation and an ever-extending notion of what constitutes dance in performance. Choreographic practice as well as research on choreography draws on new methods of improvisation, (auto-)biography, collective creation and immersion in ways which challenge established (Western) notions of subjectivity, of the artist as creator, or which unsettle the 'objective distance' between the critic and the work. The post-national, inter-medial and interdisciplinary contexts of digital and social media, festival circuits, rapidly changing political economies and global world politics call for further critical attention.

With an openness to these new worlds in which dance so adeptly manoeuvres, this book series aims to provide critical and historicised perspectives on the artists, concepts and cultures shaping this creative field of 'new world choreographies'. The series will provide a platform for fresh ways to understand and reflect upon what choreography means to its various audiences, and to the wider field of international dance and performance studies. Additionally, it will also provide a forum for new scholars to expand upon their ideas and to map out new knowledge paradigms that introduce this diverse and exciting field of choreographic practice to dance, theatre and performance studies.

Rachel Fensham
University of Melbourne
Australia

Peter M. Boenisch
Aarhus University
Denmark

Siobhan Murphy
Series Administration
Parkville, Aarhus

http://www.newworldchoreographies.com

PREFACE

I first met Sidi Larbi Cherkaoui in the autumn of 2003 in the auditorium of a municipal theatre in a provincial town in Flanders, after a performance of *Foi* (2003) and after all the other spectators had left. I had been in touch with Les Ballets C. de la B. about being introduced to Cherkaoui to speak to him about my research that I had begun to carry out about his work as part of my Master's studies at the University of Surrey. He was intrigued by the notion that someone would do research about his work. I showed him the essays I had been writing, which analysed *Rien de Rien* (2000), told him that I was considering writing my Master's dissertation about his work *Foi*, and asked him if it would be possible for me to come in and observe some of his creation process. He kindly agreed and invited me in to witness the final ten days of the creation process of *Tempus Fugit* (2004) that summer.

Since then we built a professional friendship, through which I was able to develop my research methodology of a dramaturgically engaged spectatorship. It has been a formative decade of research for me, in which I journeyed from my white, middle-class, Flemish, Catholic background to Rotterdam and then London, studying and teaching dance and interrogating my own identity, privilege, sociocultural attitudes and world views.

I think back to my childhood in a small, rural village between Brussels and Antwerp and remember the strong, clear sense of identity I had at the time. When I was seven or eight, I used to make identity cards for myself, in anticipation of my twelfth birthday, which is the age at which every Belgian citizen receives a compulsory identity card. In the meantime, my home-made card featured a small pencil drawing of my face on the left-hand side and my name and date of birth on the right. Also on the right was a list of geographical specifications: my address, my village, Antwerp province, Flanders, Belgium, Europe, the world, the universe. I clearly knew my place in the world, where I belonged, where people could find me. I visualised a world, indeed a universe, in which I was at the centre. My mother took the makeshift identity card into work and gave it permanence by laminating it for me and bringing it back home with her. Into my wallet it went, alongside paper circles for coins and fake banknotes; and so, I was playing at adulthood, which I imagined would be characterised by clarity and confidence.

We were Catholic, my family and I, like the majority of Belgians in the 1980s. We went to mass every Sunday or Saturday evening, along with my grandparents and extended family. Usually we went to our small local church, but occasionally we went to the Saint Rumbold's Cathedral in Mechelen. This impressive Gothic cathedral is recognisable from the outside by its flat-topped tower, once designed to be the highest church tower ever built, but left unfinished when the funds ran out. As a child, I had climbed the spiral staircase of the tower on a school trip. The cathedral's interior has left a deep impression on me: the high pillars leading its visitors' eyes up to heaven, the sculptures of saints, daylight filtered through the colourful stained glass windows, the emotive Baroque paintings, the deeply vibrating tones of the organ, the incense. I served a stint as an acolyte at my local church, drawn to the theatricality of the weekly ceremonies, the candles, the bread, the wine and the bells. Later, my parents and I sang in the church choir. I attended the same local, Catholic primary and secondary school as my father had. Childhood was marked by Holy Communion at age six and Confirmation at age twelve, both of which were accompanied by a big celebration, chic new clothes, fancy hairdos, photo shoots in the park, the exchange of prayer cards, and presents. I had a strong sense of belonging in this religious community. Catholicism's Gothic and Baroque iconographies, its architecture, rituals and stories have all left a strong, indelible mark on my consciousness, even if I stopped practising religion and developed atheist views in my adult life. It is only later, through travel and scholarly pursuits, that I became conscious of how deeply Western culture is permeated by Christian imagery and ways of thinking. Until then, I had never questioned that this was the expected way of being in the world. I had a faint understanding of the violence that had been carried out throughout history in the name of Christianity, crusades and colonisation, but had not approached these questions from the cultural relativism that I later adopted.

Flemish, the Dutch language spoken in Flanders, was the language we spoke at home, although we learnt French, English and German at school. Both my parents imparted a sense of Flemish nationalism on me. The stories told by my mother, originally from a Brussels suburb, illustrate the kinds of linguistic oppression she had experienced by the growing French-speaking majority there, as Flemish people were routinely stereotyped as simple, unrefined peasants. My father began his university studies at the Catholic University of Louvain in the late 1960s, around the time of the 'Leuven Vlaams' (Louvain Flemish) campaign, which fought for the linguistic separation of the University. The campaign eventually led to the Francophone branch of the University, the Université Catholique de Louvain, to be relocated to a newly built town south of the language 1962 border: Louvain-la-Neuve. In my family, there was a strong sense that the spreading of French into the Flemish territories around Brussels should be combatted, that we should be proud to speak Flemish and that, on the rare occasions we went to Brussels, we should insist that officials and shop assistants address us in Flemish, as they should be bilingual and we should not compromise our Flemish presence in the capital. At the same time as there was this defence of local culture, there was a contrasting urge that we should learn other languages, to be able to communicate with people from other countries, with our futures in global economies in mind. As a family, we visited a range of European countries on holiday: France, Italy, Austria, Germany and Spain, and took in the local languages, cultures, museums and sights, particularly the churches.

Why am I telling this story of my childhood? It is because my stable sense of national, cultural, religious and linguistic identity could not be more different from Cherkaoui's. If I am to make the argument of the dramaturgy of the spectator, or the social transformation that the spectator may go through in response to Cherkaoui's work, it is vital to understand the distance I have travelled in my own shifting world view. The most significant impact of my dramaturgical engagement with Cherkaoui's work has been that I have stopped seeing my own identity, my own body, as unmarked.

I have been following his work since 1999 as a spectator and scholar. While studying for my Master's at the University of Surrey, I undertook in-depth choreographic analysis of his works *Rien de Rien* and *Foi* from a distance, as an audience member. It was during this time, in February 2004, that I introduced myself and my M.A. research to Cherkaoui, and, as a result, was given the opportunity to carry out multiple interviews with him and other performers, and to witness intensively the final week of creation of *Tempus Fugit* in Châteauvallon, France, before it entered its premiere at the Avignon festival in July 2004. Since then, I have watched Cherkaoui's major works, some several times. At the same time, I have been prevented from seeing some of his smaller works, such as *In Memoriam* (2004), commissioned by Les Ballets de Monte Carlo, and *Orbo Novo* (2009), commissioned by Cedar Lake Contemporary Ballet, as these have not entered major touring and my resources to travel have been limited. Next, I will describe key moments taken from that period when I observed creation of new works and significant conversations with Cherkaoui and the people he works with, which have been crucial in the development of my role of engaged spectator.

In July 2004 in Châteauvallon and Avignon, I spent ten days observing the creation of *Tempus Fugit*. In the afternoons, small groups of performers worked in the studio space fine-tuning the choreographic material, independently or with Cherkaoui's guidance. Each evening was taken up by a run-through of the whole work in the outdoor performance space. The structure of the work was beginning to take shape, but still quite major alterations were made to it, most significantly in terms of the transitions between scenes and the duration of individual sections of material. The evenings were invariably concluded by a conversation with the group as a whole, in which Cherkaoui reflected on the effectiveness of the choreography and changes were suggested, to be tried out the next day. I had numerous informal conversations with Cherkaoui and the performers, unrecorded apart from in my own reflective scribbles, because the use of a voice recorder was often not appropriate in this kind of dramaturgical context. Nor was there much free time for either Cherkaoui or the collaborators to spend talking to me without interruption. In these conversations, I discussed the choreographic and dramaturgical choices made in the creation and performance of the works with him and other performers. In some instances, my feedback and ideas when watching rehearsals were welcomed and used by Cherkaoui as dramaturgical advice, probably because he performed in this work himself and valued my response as a spectator, and so I became part of the broader dramaturgical context of the work. I therefore quickly crossed the border from non-participant observer to becoming part of the fabric of collaborators. I ate with the performers, the choreography assistant, the lighting designer, technicians, sound engineer, costume designers, production manager, the person who cared for Marc Wagemans—a performer in the work who has Down's Syndrome—and other visitors, and I shared a room with the costume designer's assistant. Any illusion that my presence would not influence the creation process was quickly shattered, and in fact it was almost expected that it would. If I was going to be there, present in the rehearsal room and in daily run-throughs of the work in the evening, then I might as well help out, by sharing my interpretations of and thoughts about the potential significance of different scenes.

During my Ph.D. project, I also became involved in observing the creation of *Babel*^(words) (2010), Cherkaoui's co-creation with his long-standing collaborator Damien Jalet. I spent a week in Antwerp in the summer of 2009 to observe workshops in preparation for the creation and returned to Belgium at regular intervals to witness the creation process of this work between January and April 2010 in the building of De Munt/La Monnaie opera in Brussels. My presence was justified by being Cherkaoui's invited guest; my long-standing relationships with many of the performers; my extensive knowledge of his works; and my awareness of his artistic concerns. When I was there, I often migrated around and through the rehearsal space. I began to join in the warm-up and singing sessions, in order to gain an embodied understanding of these practices. I did not participate in the other workshop activities, primarily because my body was not sufficiently trained to cope with the virtuosic movement material, but also because I wanted to focus on note-taking as a way for me to describe and analyse my observations and experiences.

It was interesting for me to witness the very beginning of the creation period, during the two-week workshop period in July and August 2009. A large and diverse group of performers was invited to take part in the workshops, which consisted of a daily warm-up yoga session, learning some of Cherkaoui's existing choreography, improvisation and composition of new movement material around the themes Cherkaoui and Jalet wanted to explore in the work, and singing sessions led by invited musicians. These workshops also functioned as an audition, because at this time it was not yet known who would be creating and performing *Babel*$^{(words)}$. It was illuminating to see how initial ideas were translated into movement material. The outcomes of composition sessions were shared in showing moments, which were often filmed. When the creation was resumed in January 2010, it was remarkable how much of the initial material had survived. Indeed, when considering the work as it is currently performed on stage, many of the initial movement concepts have found their way into the finalised choreography. During the period from January to April 2010, the selected group of performers worked with Cherkaoui and Jalet to develop the existing material, to create new material and to work towards an overall dramaturgical structure of the work, assisted by Nienke Reehorst as choreography assistant and Lou Cope as dramaturg. My role in this process was similar to the role I had previously assumed with *Tempus Fugit* and *Myth* (2007): my exchanges with Cherkaoui, Jalet, Cope and the performers helped to develop my active engagement with the work's choreographic and dramaturgical layers and its evocative imagery. On one particular occasion in March, after rehearsals, Cherkaoui and I travelled together on the train from Brussels to Antwerp. It was a brief, unrecorded half-hour conversation, in a train carriage we shared with other passengers. Such conversations, as opposed to formal, substantial and recorded interviews, are the bread and butter of my relationship with Cherkaoui, stolen moments in busy schedules, yet no less valued. Next, I will describe a number of other significant conversations I had with Cherkaoui throughout the time I have known him.

In April 2004, I conducted my first formal interview with Cherkaoui in Antwerp as part of my Master's research on *Foi*. The interview was semi-structured and video recorded. It mainly focused on the relationship between movement and music in *Foi*, and cultural issues emerging from the work. In my questions I highlighted moments from the work that I found interesting and Cherkaoui explained how they came into being, for example, which performer had brought certain elements to the creation process from their cultural background and then how this material developed during the choreographic process. This type of conversation, minus the degree of formality, would serve as a blueprint for future conversations he and I would have. Later that year in June, *Foi* was performed in London, and I had the opportunity to talk with many of the performers involved in the creation of the work. In these audio-recorded conversations I fine-tuned my understanding of various cultural elements of the work by asking the relevant performers more detailed questions. Because I visited multiple performances of the same work, I also built a relatively durable relationship with the performers; I became a familiar face in the audience and in the bar after the show.

When I approached Cherkaoui in February 2007 about engaging in doctoral research on his work, exploring with him the possibility of holding further conversations and perhaps observing creation, I was invited to attend a preview in Antwerp, an informal sharing of work done to date, of his work *Myth*. The sharing took the shape of a showing of draft scenes and loose fragments of performance material in a provisional order. The event was attended by the co-producers of the work, most notably Guy Cassiers, the then artistic director of Het Toneelhuis, which is the municipal theatre company of Antwerp. *Myth* was the first major production Cherkaoui created under the Toneelhuis umbrella after leaving Les Ballets C. de la B. The sharing represented quite a laden moment in a new collaborative structure, in the sense that Cherkaoui allowed the Toneelhuis staff a glimpse into his new creation and welcomed their feedback. Afterwards he and I talked about the event, the feedback from his colleagues at the Toneelhuis and the artistic work itself. I realised that I had been invited to witness that sharing as Cherkaoui's friend, someone already familiar with his artistic concerns and there to offer support. In the months preceding the start of my Ph.D. research between June and October 2007 I attended the premiere and first series of performances of *Myth* in Antwerp. Following an evening tryout of the work in the theatre, Cherkaoui and I talked through my impressions and understanding of the work. I had many questions about aspects of the work derived from the diverging cultural backgrounds of the performers, and over the next few months I set about exploring these with him and the performers as I attended repeated performances of *Myth*, following this work at specific intervals from its premiere to its closing performance.

On a few occasions, I travelled to places especially to watch choreography by Cherkaoui. In April 2009, I travelled to Dublin to see the performance of *Apocrifu* (2007), a work I had not had the opportunity to see before and, I was worried, would not have the chance to see elsewhere. It was performed as part of the Dublin Dance Festival. I had a substantial informal conversation with Cherkaoui in the afternoon talking him through what I had achieved and discovered so far in my doctoral research in the months leading up to my upgrade to M.Phil. Cherkaoui responded by making links between some of the outcomes

of my performance analysis and scenes from other works which he had
created that shared similar artistic concerns. I was keen to ensure I was
not misrepresenting Cherkaoui's work in my writing, so I was mainly
checking whether he could find himself in the points I highlighted as of
interest to me in his work. On the whole, this was the case and I took
away an increased sense of confidence from the conversation. In the
evening, after seeing the performance, I was able to talk through some of
the moments from the work with Cherkaoui and the other performers,
Dimitri Jourde and Yasuyuki Shuto, who did not speak English very well
and with whom I conversed in broken French—his better than mine—
with the aid of Cherkaoui's choreography assistant Satoshi Kudo to
translate to and from Japanese. The evening was interrupted by speeches,
one of which was by the Belgian ambassador in Dublin. He had an overt
political agenda and seemed to be mobilising Cherkaoui's work, with
which he only engaged rudimentarily, for his own ambassadorial purposes. I thought this was misplaced, particularly in light of the complex
political issues in Belgium, which will be discussed in depth in Chapter 1,
the introduction to this book. This incident led me to achieve a broader
connection with Cherkaoui about the way his work was functioning as
part of a larger economic and political framework.

In June 2009, following a performance of *Sutra* (2008) at Sadler's
Wells in London, I was invited to dinner with Cherkaoui, Jalet and
Antony Gormley, who would work together on the next creation,
Babel^(words). The three men discussed the themes and issues they were
looking to explore in the work, making reference to current and historical developments in global politics. I stayed in the background for much
of this conversation, but it was extremely enlightening for me to hear
them talk about what took their interest and warranted choreographic
exploration, most notably the notion of geopolitics and the continuous
shifting of spaces. This conversation preceded my initial period observing
the creation of the work in the summer of 2009.

After the premiere of *TeZukA* (2011) in September 2011 at Sadler's
Wells, I spoke to Cherkaoui about this work, which I found to be very
complex, perhaps one the most complex works he had made thus far.
Cherkaoui was very generous with his time on this occasion, at a recep-
tion where there were many people wanting to talk to him. I like to
think that he appreciated hearing my thoughts about the work, as
a friend and supporter. By this time, I had become more confident in
making sense of my experiences as a spectator and did not pursue my

usual agenda of trying to find out answers to questions I had about the work, which I knew could come later or not at all. I realised my reading of the work would still be equally valid not knowing the answers to my questions. This realisation marked a shift in my own understanding of the engaged spectatorship methodology: it became less concerned with tracing origin or decoding and instead began to focus on excavating the imagery and iconographies within the works independently while trusting my own ability to navigate the complex, multi-layered dramaturgies as a spectator. There is thus potential for engaged spectatorship as a research methodology to extend to other spectators, who do not have the benefit of privileged access to the works' creators like I had. Repeated viewings of a work help to facilitate a deeper engagement with its dramaturgical content; this is facilitated by ready access to video recordings of the some of the works, for example *zero degrees* and *Sutra*. Without the ability to watch a work more than once, engaged spectatorship is still possible and hinges on spectators' ability to analyse choreography in the moment and articulate their insights through conversations with others after watching the performance. Discursive exchanges of this kind help spectators to remember aspects of the performance, to compare experiences, and to share in others' perspectives on the cultural aspects of the work. Engaged spectatorship is a skill that must be developed and practised, like a muscle that needs strengthening through regular exercise.

I maintain occasional email and web-based contact with some of Cherkaoui's closest collaborators, including Iris Bouche, Lou Cope, Guy Cools, Damien Fournier, Damien Jalet, Satoshi Kudo, Christine Leboutte, Karthika Naïr, Laura Neyskens and Darryl E. Woods. Throughout the years, many of these people have continued to work with Cherkaoui on other productions and I kept encountering them again and again, so they have become my friends, on Facebook. Over time, I have moved from preparing and recording each interview very carefully to a much more informal approach. This is due to my changing role in the process: I started as an outside researcher and became more of an insider, a visitor, a friend. While this could be considered problematic, I would argue that the benefits of the insider perspective, with a residue of the conversation in my reflective field notes, outweigh any perceived benefits of formalised record keeping. I have maintained a healthy relationship with the people I have spoken to, and I have no indication that they felt uncomfortable sharing their thoughts with me at any point.

This may be due to the fact that conversations mainly took place with me as a spectator, after the performances. I was less interested in unveiling the creation process, and even though I have witnessed a glimpse of the creation of some of the works, the emphasis of my research is on the work as it is performed on stage, something which is in the public domain and with which I engage as a spectator. It is in this sphere of hermeneutics that my research operates and in which I see the possibility of a dramaturgically engaged spectatorship emerging.

London, UK   Lise Uytterhoeven

ACKNOWLEDGEMENTS

First and foremost, I would like to express my deepest gratitude to Professor Rachel Fensham, who has supervised my doctoral research project since its inception, for her inspirational guidance, patience and generous encouragement. Rachel also nurtured me in developing my thesis into this book as part of the New World Choreographies series, which she co-edits with Professor Peter Boenisch. I am indebted to Peter not only for his work as series co-editor, but also for nudging along my research during a postgraduate research event at Royal Holloway and further exchanges at a TaPRA working group during the early stages of my doctorate. I would also like to give special thanks to Dr. Helena Hammond, who co-supervised my doctoral project in the beginning years, and to Dr. Efrosini Protopapa, who co-supervised the completion of my thesis in its final stages. In addition to these key mentors, I would like to thank the other staff at the University of Surrey and my peers in the Postgraduate Research community for helping to shape my research by giving feedback during the biannual Research Weeks.

The support that Sidi Larbi Cherkaoui has lent to my research over the years has been invaluable. Being a person of real kindness, generosity, positive energy and inspiration, he has provided me with generous access to his performances, creation processes and archival material and put me in touch with so many interesting people. Even when I could see he was extremely busy, he was still able to find little moments to talk to me, for which I am immensely grateful. I would also like to thank Cherkaoui's artistic collaborators who took time to speak with me about their work:

most notably Damien Jalet, Karthika Naïr, Satoshi Kudo, Christine Leboutte, Darryl E. Woods, Ulrika Kinn Svensson, Laura Neyskens, Daisy Ransom Phillips, Helder Seabra, Damien Fournier, Patrizia Bovi, Lou Cope and Guy Cools. I am also grateful to the producers and assistants at Eastman, Frans Brood Productions and Toneelhuis for providing me with the necessary schedules and logistic support. Lars Boot deserves a very special mention from me in this regard; thank you for everything.

Sincere thanks go out to my colleagues, students and graduates at London Studio Centre, and my students at University of Surrey and University Campus Suffolk (now University of Suffolk) over the past few years. I thoroughly enjoyed sharing my research findings with them in my classes and in corridor conversations, and engaging with their responses to Cherkaoui's work, which I found to be very enriching. I would like to mention my colleague Dr. Francis Yeoh in particular, because he has been an incredibly supportive sounding board with whom I could share my experiences.

I would like to thank the Arts and Humanities Research Council (AHRC) for awarding me a doctoral grant, which has allowed me to pursue my research with the necessary focus.

Finally, I would like to thank my family and friends for their encouragement and loving support. Heartfelt thanks to my father, Herman, for providing inspiration to aim high and for supporting me when the going got tough; my mother, Lucia, for helping me to translate French text and indeed for providing me with the stable family basis that has given me so much confidence; my sister, Nele, and my brother, Stijn, and my siblings-in-law, Frédéric and Astrid, for accompanying me to the theatre to watch Cherkaoui's works and for lifting my spirits; my partner, Carmelo, for his endless love and encouragement that inspired me to finish both my thesis and complete this book; my family-in-law, Angela, Salvatore and Tanina, for the support, home-cooked meals and child-care which gave me precious time to devote to writing the book; and my daughter, Mia, for brightening my days with singing, lovely cuddles and smiles.

I am beyond grateful to my friends and colleagues for all our exchanges about the project and life in general: in alphabetic order, Naomi Barber, Katelijne Bax, Melissa Blanco Borelli, Sue Booker, Luke Brown, Sarahleigh Castelyn, Broderick Chow, Fiona Compton, Deveril, Mike Dixon, Sherril Dodds, Moe Dodson, Kathrina Farrugia-Kriel, Rachel Forster, Liam Francis, Kurt Frooninckx, Hannah Gibbs, Julia K. Gleich,

Bianca Greenhalgh, Joanna Hall, Nesreen Nabil Hussein, Jennifer Jackson, Louise Kelsey, Sarah Kerr, Anuradha Kowtha, Josephine Leask, Chih-Chieh Liu, Yael Loewenstein, Kathy Milazzo, Dara Milovanonic, Royona Mitra, Celena Monteiro, Jay O'Shea, Josh Owen, Clare Parfitt-Brown, Robert Penman, Daniela Perazzo Domm, Stacey Prickett, Prarthana Purkayastha, Laura Robinson, Maria Salgado Llopis, Lucia Schweigert, Sabine Sörgel, Victoria Thoms, Katalin Trencsényi, Tim Trimingham Lee, Florent Trioux, Laura Weston, Esther Willett and Manrutt Wongkaew.

CONTENTS

LIST OF FIGURES

CHAPTER 1

Introduction—Kaleidoscopic Identity and Aesthetics

Since his choreographic debut in 1999 for Les Ballets C. de la B., Flemish-Moroccan dance theatre choreographer Sidi Larbi Cherkaoui has become a prolific creator of new works in a variety of contexts, including *Rien de Rien* (2000), *Foi* (2003), *zero degrees* (co-choreographed with Akram Khan, 2005), *Myth* (2007), *Apocrifu* (2007), *Sutra* (2008) and *Babel^(words)* (co-choreographed with Damien Jalet, 2010). These works, made in the first decade of the new millennium, and the processes that yielded them, are characterised by cross-cultural collaboration and onstage complexity. In this book, I will articulate and analyse the challenges presented for spectators in these staged works and argue that the labour in which spectators are invited to engage is dramaturgical in nature.

Before introducing Cherkaoui through the perhaps conventional biographical approach, a more exciting starting point rooted in choreographic analysis is *La Zon-Mai* (2007), a three-dimensional multimedia art installation for museums and gallery spaces in the shape of a house, co-created by choreographer Sidi Larbi Cherkaoui and film-maker Gilles Delmas. From the inside of the house, moving images are projected on its white walls and roof, snippets of film capturing 21 dancers moving in their homes across Paris, London, Berlin, Vienna, Wellington, Tokyo and Buenos Aires. These dancers are among Cherkaoui's closest friends, who have given shape to his choreographic productions thus far. This work, not conceived for the stage but equally intent on storytelling through choreography, honours some of Cherkaoui's closest collaborators in the

© The Author(s) 2019
L. Uytterhoeven, *Sidi Larbi Cherkaoui*, New World Choreographies,
https://doi.org/10.1007/978-3-030-27816-8_1

2000–2010 period. If nothing else, it is through an understanding of his unstoppable collaborative and transcultural drive, a drive to connect with others across cultures, that his choreographic project crystallises in the observer's mind.

INTERSECTIONS BETWEEN HOME, PLACE AND IDENTITY IN *LA ZON-MAI*

A spectator writes: 'One dancer hops along her kitchen worktop, curled up like a foetus. Another spins dizzyingly on a living room rug. Yet another performs a remarkable bathroom ballet between the toilet and the washbasin' (Stevens). Another reviewer recalls: 'Akram Khan [...] dances in his narrow foyer, spinning tightly within its confines. Shantala Shivalingappa's arms can't cut through the glass doors to her balcony. A contortionist in green gym shorts tears up his living room floor. A dancer with long black hair combed over her face slices through the veil with her hands' (Jackson). The films are projected in a loop on a house-shaped building without doors and windows, without ever physically allowing the viewer to step through its threshold. Walking around the installation in the museum or gallery space, the spectator encounters these intimate films of dancers in their homes accompanied by a moving soundtrack of medieval and traditional songs, arranged by Vladimir Ivanoff (Fig. 1.1).

La Zon-Mai was commissioned by the Cité National de l'Histoire de l'Immigration in Paris, as part of a project aiming to change the perception of, and prejudices towards, immigration (Cherkaoui & Delmas). The Cité is housed in the former Musée des Colonies et de la France Extérieure. The irony of this remarkable metamorphosis of the building's purpose does not escape Cherkaoui.

> A place dedicated to colonialism has been dug up to allow the nation to pay homage to the phenomenon of immigration! [...] I found this fascinating, troubling and at the same also typically French: the ability to overturn these roles and to confront the present with the past. (Cherkaoui & Delmas 9)

La Zon-Mai was conceived to be placed at the centre of the Festival Hall of the Palais de la Porte Dorée, a room adorned with colonial frescoes depicting the radiation of French culture across the world.

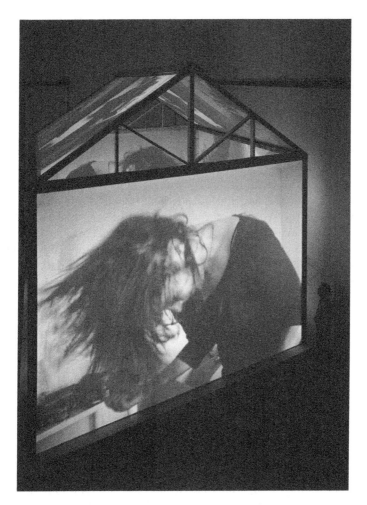

Fig. 1.1 *La Zon-Mai*, multimedia installation created by Sidi Larbi Cherkaoui and Gilles Delmas (Photo by Gilles Delmas)

These frescoes are based on the ethnocentric, colonial paradigm, in which Europe proclaimed itself the centre of the world and regarded the cultures it encountered as Other, 'à l'extérieur'. In contrast, in Cherkaoui's philosophy 'one is never at the centre and always exists in reference to something else' (2007 Interview). Thus, he is interested in 'a process of learning to think, to travel whilst decentring oneself, without considering oneself as the pivot' (Cherkaoui & Delmas 10). In response to the overturning of the building's concept and purpose, *La Zon-Mai* is shaped as an inside-out house. What goes on behind closed doors is readily visible here, projected onto the exterior walls, the private made public. The dance films echo the frescoes on the walls of the room; these animated frescoes are described by Cherkaoui as 'an intimate cartography' and 'a precious family album', as these dancers form part of what he calls 'his personal story/history [in French "histoire"]' (Cherkaoui & Delmas 23).

This inversion of inside and outside is mirrored in the work's title by the reversal of the syllables of the French word for 'house' or 'home' ('maison'/'zon-mai'). Inverting syllables is characteristic of Verlan, a French language game and secret language turned slang. In response to Cherkaoui's dramaturgical interest in language as symptomatic for larger cultural issues, the methodologies used in my research on Cherkaoui's work draw heavily on theories of language, particularly translation studies and theorisations of storytelling. In the case of *La Zon-Mai*, too, sociological perspectives on language immediately shine an interesting light on the title of this installation. From second-generation North-African immigrants in the Parisian *banlieue* who describe themselves as 'les beurs' (Verlan for 'les arabes'), Verlan has been appropriated into 'le parler d'jeunes', youth speak in general and has become a common occurrence in hip hop music. Verlan has, for a considerable time indeed, been 'penetrating the rigid boundaries of Standard Modern French' (Lefkowitz 2). The use of the sociolect Verlan could be read as an act of undermining the hegemonic qualities of the French language, the language of colonisation. The Verlan word 'zon-mai' is an attack on the concept of 'home' itself, which for the second-generation immigrants in Paris has gone topsy-turvy. Cherkaoui was born and grew up in Antwerp, Belgium, as the son of a Moroccan father and a Flemish mother. Being both second generation and culturally 'mixed', his sense of belonging and identity has never been unambiguous or straightforward. By Verlanising the word for house/home, Cherkaoui and Delmas do more than merely aligning themselves with marginalised youth subcultures. Verlanisation shows that languages themselves, and by extension cultures at large, are dynamic and ever-changing, never static or fixed.

More recent research on Verlan has paid attention to deeper ethnographic understandings of its role in the construction of identity. Verlan is framed as 'a social practice through which youths can position themselves in relation to their peers and to the dominant discourse in a variety of ways' (Doran 101). Ginette Vincendeau, a film scholar specialising in popular French cinema, understands Verlan to be a marker of identity, of otherness, both dangerous/illicit and playful. Its use stresses a sense of cohesion against the outside world (Vincendeau 26), while a term such as 'beur' simultaneously erases difference. This ethnographic research highlights that Verlan is used 'to construct and participate in an alternative social sphere, in which hybrid identities – ones that did not correspond to the mono[-lingual or monocultural] norms of the hegemonic imagined community – could find expression and validation' (Doran 104). The sociolinguist Meredith Doran concludes that its use situates identity in local, second-generation communities, rather than in any particular nation. Doran continues to write that 'In terms of language, this sense of multi-ness was signalled in part by the incorporation of borrowings from family and other minority languages [...]. The heteroglossia of youths' local code serves as a means of indexing their ties to (and solidarity with) a variety of languages and cultures, allowing them to express their own sense of cultural and linguistic hybridity, tied both to France as a literal home, and to other cultures within and outside it' (Doran 111). In Chapter 5 of this book, I focus on the heteroglossia in Cherkaoui's work, in which multiple languages are spoken on stage without translation. With the aid of translation studies, this dramaturgy of non-translation is read as postcolonial critique. It is interesting to highlight this continuous heteroglossia even within the sociolect of Verlan itself, avoiding any notion of singularity and fixity.

A populariser of Verlan in mainstream music is the Belgian singer Stromae (Verlan for 'maestro'), who has won international success with his electro-hip hop sound and shares with Cherkaoui a strong historical and postcolonial awareness. Cherkaoui and Stromae were both named in a 2014 list of '25 most influential allochthonous Belgians', along with the then Belgian Prime Minister Elio Di Rupo and footballer Vincent Kompany. This problematic term, the obverse of 'autochthonous', is commonly used in Flanders to refer to non-indigenous people and is indicative of the failings of multiculturalism in Belgium and the associated rise of the populist radical right in Flanders. In recent years, the word has been problematised by some mainstream newspapers, calling for its use to be discontinued. Controversially, to mark the 50th anniversary of the arrangements made by Belgium with Morocco and Turkey for these countries to provide guest labourers, the magazine *Knack* invited a panel of academics and other experts to compile a list of 'those people of allochthonous origin in our country who have the most power and influence' (Renard & De Ceulaer). Cherkaoui's response to this 'honour' was carefully considered and very interesting. In his regular blog for *MO Magazine*, he argues for a reframing of the way the term 'allochthonous' is used.

> It is not a matter of being one or the other, not allochthonous OR Flemish, but allochthonous AND Flemish AND Antwerpian. Otherwise the word is a way to keep someone at the side line, rather than letting the person belong to the mainstream. [...] Only then [when used in conjunction with, rather than in opposition to, terms indexing other dimensions of national identity] is the use of a word like "allochthonous" responsible, or even – and that would be nice – enriching in the cultural exchange process. (Cherkaoui *MO Magazine*)

Eschewing the pitfalls of dichotomous thinking and the power issues that come with it, Cherkaoui calls for a firm embracing of identity as plural and intersectional. Given that there is no direct equivalent in the English language of 'allochthonous' as it is used to denote otherness in the Flemish sociopolitical and media context, I have opted to include this controversial, even jarring, term from time to time in this book. Without wishing to maintain or support the underpinning dichotomies between 'nationally-identified indigenous' and 'foreigner/immigrant/ethnic', my echoing of its use by cultural commentators on Cherkaoui's work serves to highlight the deeper sociopolitical attitudes with which his work has been approached and considered in the Flemish collective imagination.

Returning to the brief Cherkaoui was given by the Cité in response to its mission, in his collaboration with Delmas for *La Zon-Mai*, Cherkaoui wanted to 'show how cultures have always been closely linked, how everything is in constant mutation, and show that there is constant natural migration. I wanted to put to the fore how much of the movement that consists of going from one place to another, from one country to another, is natural' (qtd. in Hervé 24). Of course, Cherkaoui does not want to brush over the significantly diverging nature of people's experiences and emphasises that migration is a complex issue. By no means can the experience of a professional dancer who moves to another country to exercise his profession be equated to that of someone who has had to leave his home country because of military conflict, poverty or political oppression.

> There are as many definitions of immigration as there are immigrants. Some miss their country of origin, others have forgotten it. Some have left their family there, others have built one in the place where they ended up. Whether it is political, sentimental or professional, both a collective and personal history/story uniquely taint the immigration experience. [...] What binds all these people who have had to leave one day is an intensive search for a home. (Cherkaoui & Delmas 24)

'There was also a strong desire to address the notion of "home", in order to remember that there are different ways of envisaging this word' (Cherkaoui & Delmas 11). Literary criticism of postcolonial literature pays much attention to representations of 'home' (George) and their implications for the construct of the nation and nationalism. When thinking about home in relation to Cherkaoui, the so-called spatial turn in diaspora studies in the early 1990s provides a useful frame. Notions of essential territorial belonging are avoided, and the focus is redirected from 'roots', or a clinging on to disrupted sense of nationhood, to 'routes', or pathways (Clifford; Gilroy). Yet, home is something that is made and desired. The sociologist Avtar Brah, in *Cartographies of Diaspora: Contesting Identities,* frames the concept of 'homing desire' in reference to diasporic experiences as the construction of home through cultural practices out of a strong yearning to feel at home, somewhere. Brah explains that 'the homing desire [...] is not the same as the desire for a "homeland"' (Brah 197), as not all diasporans share the desire to return to a place of 'origin'. For second-generation migrants, of which Cherkaoui is one, the ancestral homeland remains a myth that can never be attained. The choreographer's interest in the notion of home, what his friends' homes look like and how they move in them, is an artistic exploration of homing desire, not the desire to return.

Due to delays to the refurbishing of the Festival Hall of the Palais de la Porte Dorée, *La Zon-Mai* could not be shown in the place that had inspired its existence, the frescoed room. Forced to migrate to other spaces in the Cité, the installation began to serve as its nomadic ambassador as it then also travelled to other museums in Bordeaux, Roubaix,

Bruges (where I encountered it in December 2007), Mannheim and Philadelphia. This sense of the nomadic resonates with Cherkaoui and his dance collaborators shown in the film projections. The funding of the key Belgian choreographers' work happens through a far-reaching system of international co-production, which implies that the works themselves, and their performers, engage in large international tours. Cherkaoui joined a transnational elite community of performers while studying at Anne Teresa De Keersmaeker's contemporary dance school P.A.R.T.S. (Performing Arts Research and Training Studios) in Brussels in the late nineties, and working with Les Ballets C. de la B., initially as a performer (in Alain Platel's *Iets op* Bach, 1998) and later as a choreographer. Becoming a member of a transnational artistic community provided a tangible alternative to the xenophobia experienced growing up in Antwerp in the eighties and nineties amidst the rise of the Flemish populist radical right. As a result, travelling around the world to perform and create became Cherkaoui's daily, lived artistic practice.

Moreover, he seeks out collaborative partners, dancers, co-choreographers, musicians, designers, from in- and outside of Europe. 'I work with dancers from the four corners of the globe, who constantly move [in French, self-reflexively, "se déplacent", or "displace themselves"] from one place to the next to rehearse, dance or live. Questions of movement and migration form an integral part of my existence' (Cherkaoui 2007 Interview). Cherkaoui is interested in working with these particular dancers because they have a destabilised sense of self due to a mixed cultural background or due to migration. *La Zon-Mai* places these dancers, their lives and experiences, at the centre of attention. In the films, the dancers are represented on screen with an ethnographic sensibility as they engage in poetic exploration of the notion of home as agents in the subversion of Eurocentrism. Khan is seen practising Kathak in his parents' house next to the washing machine, holding an iPod and wearing earphones. The dancers' affective, post-Fordist and transnational dance labour and fluid identities are mobilised by Cherkaoui and Delmas against the idea of nation and empire.

In sum, both in its spatial design, its filmic and choreographic subject matter, and in its title, *La Zon-Mai* is deeply infused with biography and ethnography. The work is read here as a postcolonial critique of conceptions of the world according to notions of centre and periphery, and part of a larger deterritorialisation project aiming to divorce culture from place.

LIVING AND WORKING IN A BELGIAN CONTEXT OF FEDERAL INSTABILITY AND POLITICAL IMPASSE

Cherkaoui was born on 10 March 1976, in Antwerp. Until the age of twelve, he attended Qur'an school under his father's influence (Cherkaoui *Curriculum Vitae*). However, he experienced a difficult relationship with his father, whose beliefs were incompatible with his adolescent views. At age fifteen, his father disappeared from his life, and Cherkaoui never sought contact with him again. In 1996, aged 20, Cherkaoui began his career as a successful dancer/choreographer. In this same year, his father died of a stroke (Cherkaoui *Curriculum Vitae*). The influence of religion plays a significant role in his artistic work, while he also negotiates his complex cultural positioning. Being of mixed origin and having a Moroccan name while growing up in Flanders, Cherkaoui has always found it difficult to fully identify with a single culture. In Antwerp during the late 1980s and early 1990s, Cherkaoui witnessed the rise of the populist radical right Vlaams Blok/Belang (VB) party, which brought many issues of national identity to the forefront that converged within his own hybrid background. These political developments took place within a fragile Belgian state.

For the duration of my doctoral research (2007–2012) on which this book is based, which roughly coincided with the works Cherkaoui made in the latter half of the 2000–2010 decade, Belgian politics was characterised by significant instability and impasse. The government formation after the federal elections of 10 June 2007, won by the Flemish cartel CD&V (Christian Democratic party)/N-VA (New Flemish Alliance), took 194 days and involved five different political figures passing through the role of appointed negotiator. The precariously formed government, led by Yves Leterme and inaugurated on 21 December 2007, fell on 22 April 2010 after Alexander De Croo, the Liberal party leader deserted the government after the issue of splitting the electoral arrondissement Brussels-Halle-Vilvoorde (BHV) remained unresolved. New elections followed on 13 June 2010, this time convincingly won by the N-VA, led by Bart De Wever, on the Dutch-speaking side and the PS (Walloon Socialist Party), led by Di Rupo, on the French-speaking side. However, the differences between these two parties from either side of the language border seemed insurmountable and metonymically began to stand for the differences between Flanders and Wallonia in general. Painfully complex and protracted negotiations followed for approximately 18 months, which saw ten different negotiators take charge of the formation process. Due to the significant problems with the government formation, many voices in the domestic and international press expressed concern about whether this political impasse signalled the end of Belgium. This section examines the historical development of this federal instability in Belgium.

After decades of debates since the 1960s and several stages of reform in 1970, 1980, 1988–1989, 1993 and 2001, the Belgian state is currently a federal state, composed of different communities and regions whose territories partly overlap. The Belgian state consists of three cultural/linguistic communities—Dutch-speaking, French-speaking and German-speaking—and three geographic regions—Flanders, Wallonia and the bilingual Brussels-Capital region. The public law scholar Patrick Peeters identifies the underlying reason for the perceived 'Belgian problem' to be the coexistence of a majority of Dutch-speaking people in the northern part of the country, Flanders, against a minority of French-speakers in the southern part, Wallonia and a small minority of German speakers near the eastern border with Germany (Peeters 32). Interestingly, the Brussels-Capital Region is dominated by a Francophone majority and the Dutch-speaking community occupies a minority position there. This problem has historically been tackled within the framework of a single Belgian state through a process of federalisation, which is devolutionary rather than integrative. The term centrifugality is used to indicate this increased transfer of powers from the central level to that of the communities and regions. The major political parties, namely the Catholics, Liberals, Socialists and Greens, have been divided into separate Flemish and Francophone parties, severely complicating governmental decision-making processes (Peeters 'Multinational Federations').

The bipolarity of the federation continues to present significant problems for resolving issues and on many occasions even for forming a government. Belgian politics is often an object of mockery in the international media, for example at the time of the record-breaking duration of government formation in 2010 and the street celebrations that followed in Belgium's major cities, labelled 'La Revolución de Patatas Fritas' in Spanish media, or 'The Chips Revolution'. Young people took off their clothes in public and partied in the streets to celebrate Belgium's sinister honour of holding the world record. An earlier performative act aiming to stir up debate about 'the Belgian problem' also did not go unnoticed in the international media. The fictional documentary, *Bye Bye Belgium*, by the Walloon national television station RTBF in December 2006, staging the end of the Belgian state after Flemish nationalists had allegedly proclaimed the independence of Flanders, illustrated that the situation is sensitive. Many people on both sides of the language border believed the fictive reports to be true, causing a short-lived panic until the programme makers subtitled the images with 'Ceci est une fiction' ('This is fiction'). This caption reminisces René Magritte's surrealist painting of a pipe, subtitled with 'Ceci n'est pas une pipe'. The fictional documentary may have been intended as a joke to alleviate tensions or may have had the aim of stimulating dialogue on the topic; however, for the international and national public the act of 'staging' the dissolution of the nation had merely added to the confusion.

Historically, the Belgian state used to exemplify a 'consociational democracy', referring to a 'government by elite cartel to turn a democracy with a fragmented political culture into a stable democracy'; however, during the first decade of the new millennium, stability seemed far out of reach (Deschouwer 895). This was playfully demonstrated in an interactive game that could be played on the website of the newspaper *De Standaard* following the June 2010 elections, entitled 'Form your own coalition', in which readers could click on the parties they would like to include in their coalition, displaying each selected party's seat representation in a different colour in a pie chart and offering feedback on the selection (Bossuyt & De Lobel). This offered readers insight into the many requirements of government formation in the Belgian consociational democracy: the selected coalition should represent a majority on both the Flemish and the Walloon sides and should have the overall two-thirds majority required to effectuate a new reformation of the Belgian state. Coalitions without French-speaking parties were thus 'not workable' (Bossuyt & De Lobel). Any pie chart that met the requirements resembled a rainbow consisting of no less than five parties.

Imagery of fracture permeates the representation of the conflict in the domestic media. Geopolitically, the language border divides Belgian in half and assigns certain territory to the respective regions and communities. However, this imagery has recently been nuanced by emphasising that the country will not so easily be divided as Belgian cartography suggests. A cartoon depiction in *De Standaard* newspaper showed the shape of Belgium, in which the different parts are held together with screws, stitches and glue, suggesting that the sense of unity is fragile (Sturtewagen). The paper also published a series of drawings by a group of ten- to twelve-year-old children as a response to the political situation, called 'The crisis through children's eyes'. Many of the drawings included the two key political figures and winners of the 2010 election, De Wever and Di Rupo. A drawing by the ten-and-a-half-year-old Ibrahim shows De Wever as a green-tinged Hulk-like figure desperately trying to tear up the Belgian flag, with the caption 'Come on, why won't this tear?' (De Standaard). The imagery and the discourse around the political instability were infused by the signs of fracture; yet these images also demonstrated an understanding of Belgium as unbreakable or untearable.

In an article entitled 'Persistent nonviolent conflict with no reconciliation: the Flemish and Walloons in Belgium', Professor of Law at Harvard, Robert Mnookin, and Professor of Law at the Universities of Leuven and Tilburg, Alain Verbeke, explore the deep-rooted Belgian political impasse by drawing a suggestive analogy with a married couple considering a divorce. The main argument of the article is that the complex Belgian federal system is at once reflective of and instrumental in negotiating day-to-day life for these two distinct language communities. 'Today the long-standing language cleavage between the Flemish and the Francophones has been embedded into a federal structure of mind-boggling complexity that both reflects and reinforces the organisation of political, social, and cultural life on the basis of language' (Mnookin & Verbeke 153). The paradox discussed here entails that 'federal structures allowing for decentralised decision-making may exacerbate centrifugal forces and hasten the eventual breakup of the nation' (Mnookin & Verbeke 154). Question marks should be placed around the use of the term 'nation' here, because others have argued that Belgium could be more appropriately defined as a multinational state, rather than encompassing a single, unified Belgian nation (Seymour; Tierney). Mnookin and Verbeke also concede that the Belgian sense of national identity is overtly constructed, as a result of a relatively recently (1830s) engineered 'arranged marriage', and weak overall (155). There is not much glue to bind the Flemish and Walloons together, apart from a common pragmatism in seeking out workable compromise and a distrust of government and authority in general, and other anecdotal quirks involving chocolate, beer, chips and the Belgian football team, the Red Devils.

On the role of Europe in this conflict, Mnookin and Verbeke explain that, while European integration has given more powers to the different regions in Belgium, for example in matters pertaining to the environment and agriculture, it simultaneously strengthens the federal government in its policymaking responsibilities due to the need for a unified Belgian position. In their discussion of the absence of violence in the Belgian conflict, Mnookin and Verbeke identify a number of reasons as to why this may be the case: geographically, there is little day-to-day contact between Flemish and Walloons; the conflict is not seen as existential or jeopardising people's identity; historically, there are no memories of violence between the two groups; economically, Belgium remains a wealthy country; and finally, politically the complex federal structure enables the two groups to exist alongside each other, albeit in a highly inefficient and frustrating system. The most likely future of the Belgian state, according to Mnookin and Verbeke, will again be 'some sort of Belgian compromise': 'the francophone political elite will eventually, reluctantly accept some additional devolution as necessary in order to save the country', while 'the Flemish elite will get far less devolution than they desire' (179). However, a real divorce is highly unlikely.

THE FLEMISH POPULIST RADICAL RIGHT

In Belgian politics since the 1970s, the Flemish populist radical right increasingly gained in popularity until the end of the first decade of the new millennium. This nationalist movement argues for an independent Flemish state, but displays xenophobia in its attitude towards foreigners and non-European immigrants. Cherkaoui, the son of a Moroccan immigrant and raised both Catholic and Muslim, was confronted with the xenophobia and Islamophobia embedded in the Flemish populist radical right. Having formed an understanding of the complex structure of the Belgian state and some of the problems that arise from this structure in the previous section, we will take a closer look in this section at the rise of the Flemish populist radical right. This movement, it will be explained, grew out of the Flemish Movement, which has been fighting for the recognition of Flemish language and culture since the nineteenth century.

The problem of decision-making, inherent in the structure of the Belgian state, is illustrated in the lack of an overarching policy on how to manage a multicultural society. Social scientists Hassan Bousetta and

Dirk Jacobs have identified that multiculturalism has been a recurring issue in Belgian politics and society since the 1970s. The multicultural society in Belgium is considered to be the result of the 'recruitment of a temporary foreign labour force' of mostly Moroccan, Turkish and Italian labourers (Bousetta & Jacobs 23). Since the 1980s, non-European asylum seekers also form a significant ethnic minority in Belgium (Mudde *Populist Radical Right*). Multiculturalism not only refers to a situation in which culturally distinct groups coexist under post-migration or postcolonial circumstances; it also offers a specific model for the management of cultural diversity.

> In so far as monocultural states are the exception rather than the rule, multiculturalism is a reality for most countries in the world. [...] the key question [...] is that of [...] recognition in the public space [...] of particular identity differences of minority groups. (Bousetta & Jacobs 24)

'The logic of pragmatism and consensus', as a result of the multinational and mosaic nature of the Belgian state and its 'complex decision-making procedures devised to pacify [...] tensions', characterises how issues with the management of cultural diversity in the public space are dealt with on an ad hoc basis (Bousetta & Jacobs 28). The Belgian multicultural debate is limited by this non-decisive, compromising and pragmatic approach. Towards the end of the twentieth century, however, the discourse became more sharp and radical, 'heavily challenging the [...] ideal of a society where difference is mutually enriching' (Bousetta & Jacobs 23). This coincided with a steep growth of the populist radical right Vlaams Blok/Vlaams Belang (VB)[1] party since the late 1980s until 2009. In that year, the centre-right and pro-European Nieuw-Vlaamse Alliantie (N-VA, New Flemish Alliance) party stunted the growth of the VB.

Both the VB and the N-VA have their roots in the Flemish Movement, which, from the movement's inception in the nineteenth century, was originally concerned with 'the emancipation of the Dutch language (i.e. Flemish) and culture from the dominance of French speaking Belgium' (Mudde *Ideology* 81). Political scientist Cas Mudde identifies that, during the First World War, the linguistic discrimination Flemish soldiers in the Belgian army received at the hands of their fellow French-speaking officers contributed to a shift in orientation in the Flemish Movement. Following the First World War, anti-Belgian demands for a politically autonomous Flanders grew stronger.

During the Second World War, a fraction of the Flemish Movement attempted to achieve this goal through collaboration with the Nazi occupiers, and by fighting communism on the Eastern Front. After the war, repressive measures were taken against collaborators. 'Under the sway of the democratisation movement of May 1968' the political party of the Flemish Movement, the Volksunie (People's Union, VU) assumed a more left-liberal, moderately nationalist stance 'to ensure that it was regarded as a respectable coalition partner' (Mudde *Ideology* 84). In 1977, the VU signed the Egmont-pact, which launched the federalisation of Belgium. Although the Egmont-pact failed due to Flemish disagreement, by 1980 the country was

> [...] divided into three autonomous regions (Flanders, Walloon and Brussels) and into two communities, the Dutch and French speaking. Both communities could implement their own policies in the Brussels region. (Mudde *Ideology* 84)

The fact that 'Brussels had become an autonomous region of its own, instead of being an integral part of Flanders' was unacceptable for the more radical membership of the VU party, who splintered off and, at first, founded a number of new parties that later became united in 1978 under the name Vlaams Blok (Flemish Block) (Mudde *Ideology* 84).

The VB's ideological programme is based on Flemish nationalism, rejecting the multinational Belgian state and arguing for an independent Flemish state, to include any previously 'frenchified' territories. However, under the leadership of Gerolf Annemans, Filip Dewinter and Frank Vanhecke, the VB became a populist radical right party. Xenophobia characterises the way foreigners, especially non-European immigrants, are perceived as a threat. This is in line with nativist ideology, 'which holds that states should be inhabited exclusively by members of the native group [...] and that nonnative elements are fundamentally threatening to the homogeneous nation-state' (Mudde *Populist Radical Right* 19). It should, however, be understood that both nativeness and non-nativeness are determined subjectively; they are imagined constructs and often contested. Within the populist radical right ideology of the VB, there is a strong emphasis on moral values and law and order. People who are seen as deviant, such as homosexuals, drug addicts and those who are in receipt of social benefits without a valid reason are considered undesirable.

The VB is also considered a populist party, because it considers 'society to be ultimately separated into [...] "the pure people" versus "the corrupt elite"' (Mudde *Populist Radical Right* 23). The national elites are considered to have been responsible for mass immigration, which is seen as a conspiracy of the left-wing parties, trade unions and big business. The media are seen to be part of the conspiracy and under 'left-wing control'. The populist ideology also dictates that politics should be 'an expression of the *volonté générale* (general will) of the people' (Mudde *Populist Radical Right* 23). During the late 1990s, the Dutroux-affair became one of the most notable scandals of Belgian politics and society, revealing a series of judicial failures following the atrocious paedophile murders committed by Marc Dutroux. Masses of people participated in 'White Marches', demonstrating the general public's protest against the failures of the criminal justice system and the alleged cover up by a range of Belgian politicians. The VB saw in this occasion an opportunity to reinforce their attack on the Belgian government and the so-called weak law and order policies.

Since the mid-1980s until the late 2000s, the VB's ideological programme increasingly appealed to a growing number of Flemish voters. Following a fierce campaign using the new slogans 'Eigen volk eerst!' ('Own people first!') and 'Grote kuis!' ('The big clean!'), the VB party achieved overwhelming successes in the 1987 election and the 1988 local election in Antwerp. This first slogan refers to the perceived unbalanced economic situation where money is seen to be transferred from the financially stronger Flemish region to the French-speaking part, which is plagued by a higher unemployment rate. It also refers to the alleged profiting by unemployed immigrants, who are the objects to be removed from Flanders in the second slogan. The VB more than trebled its 1987 share of the vote in the parliamentary election of 24 November 1991, which was later referred to as 'Black Sunday'. Not only did the party win in large cities such as Antwerp, it also gained votes in small 'villages with no foreign inhabitants' due to the effects of its politics of fear (Mudde *Ideology* 89). During the 1990s and 2000s, the VB continued to book successes in local as well as regional and federal parliamentary elections. By 1999, the VB had become Flanders' third largest party, and in the June 2004 federal elections, it secured 25% of the popular vote.

Reasons for the continued growth of the extreme-right in Flanders appear to be the increased sense that, due to the perceived criminality of non-European immigrants, the cities are unsafe, and that the recent developments of uncontrolled immigration have an anti-Flemish effect. There are two underlying dimensions to populist radical right ideology, which are of interest to this discussion of Cherkaoui's work: Islamophobia, a fear of Islam and Muslims, and globaphobia, a fear of globalisation. The VB emphasises 'the alleged incompatibility of Islam with the basic tenets of [...] European [...] culture' (Mudde *Populist Radical Right* 85). The growth of the populist radical right in Belgium has been linked to a politics of fear. International developments that may have exacerbated this politics of fear include the terrorist attacks on the World Trade Center in New York City and other landmarks on the USA mainland on 11 September 2001, 'the war in Iraq, the Israeli-Palestinian conflict and the unstable situation in Afghanistan', which can all be seen to have 'contributed to a mutual lack of confidence between "the West" and "the Arab-Muslim world"' (Bousetta & Jacobs 24). It should, however, be acknowledged that, as a consequence of 9/11 and the 'war on terrorism', Islamophobia is not 'an exclusive feature of the populist radical right, but reaches deep into the political mainstream of most Western countries' (Mudde *Populist Radical Right* 84).

Another trait of the populist radical right is 'globaphobia', a fear of globalisation, which is seen to 'threaten the independence and purity of the nation-state' (Mudde *Populist Radical Right* 196). Ryan asserts that because Belgium has always been at the forefront of European integration, 'it is difficult to think of any other society where the impact of globalization has been so significant' (146). Cultural globalisation, or Americanisation or 'Cocacolonization', the latter term coined by the VB, 'is rejected because it is believed to annihilate the cultural diversities of nations' (Mudde *Populist Radical Right* 191–196). However, the effects of globalisation on the workings of the world in terms of migration, culture, trade, media and military intervention are so complex and full of paradoxes that they cannot be reduced to a simple slogan to be wielded for populist purposes. Hardly any explicit reference is made to globalisation in populist radical right propaganda, so that:

> by largely ignoring (though not denying) globalization, they do not have to address the question whether mass immigration and loss of sovereignty *can be* countered in the era of globalization. (Mudde *Populist Radical Right* 197)

However, another important reason is that for many people there is no other opportunity to express their dissatisfaction and frustration with the coalition of numerous mainstream political parties than to vote for the VB. This pattern of voting is referred as *foert-stem* ('sod it!-vote'). The fact that voting is a compulsory civil duty in Belgium, a situation which is contested by many, contributes to this trend. Since 1989, other Flemish parties have been debating, and eventually agreed upon, the maintenance of a *cordon sanitaire*, which translates as 'quarantine line' and refers to an unwritten agreement not to negotiate or form a coalition with the VB in order to contain the spread of its ideology, thereby excluding them from executive power and keeping them in permanent opposition. The cordon sanitaire affirms the frustration of the *foert-stemmers* ('sod it!-voters') as it has instilled a sense of being ignored and silenced by the traditional parties. The cordon sanitaire is highly controversial and heavily disputed by political scientists due to its undemocratic effect. It was expected that, in theory, the VB would lose a substantial number of votes if it did get a chance to participate in government and its manifesto would turn out to be undeliverable. However, this has now become a moot point due to the displacement of the Flemish nationalist vote to the more centre-right N-VA since 2009, which decimated the VB and brought its rise to power to a halt. The N-VA, which had soaked up a large contingent of VB voters in 2009 but is not subject to the *cordon sanitaire*, has been part of coalition governments in the Flemish parliament since 2004 and the federal parliament since 2014. The VB party has become less relevant, and—with it—the need for the *cordon sanitaire*.

Finally, it becomes possible to tie together reflections on how Belgian federal instability, political impasse and the Flemish populist radical right have influenced each other in the period under scrutiny (mid-1980s to late 2000s). Belgium's complex federal structure, in which political power is spread over multi-party 'rainbow' coalitions, fragile and time-bound, is usually regarded as inefficient and frustrating, typical of the country's non-decisive, compromising and pragmatic approach devised to pacify tensions between the two major language communities (Mnookin & Verbeke). However, together with the *cordon sanitaire* around the VB party—in other words, the other parties' refusal to form coalitions with the VB—the mosaic complexity of Belgium's political system has helped to keep populist radical right ideology at bay. This is the complex political equation during which both Cherkaoui and I came to maturity in Flanders.

CHERKAOUI'S PROLIFIC OEUVRE

Cherkaoui started his dance career in variety and television shows in Belgium, which can be considered an unconventional entry into the field of theatrical dance. In 1995, he received the first prize for the 'Best Belgian Dance Solo' in Ghent, in a competition launched by Platel of Les Ballets C. de la B.

> Encouraged by Marie-Louise Wilderijkx, his ballet teacher in Antwerp, [...] Cherkaoui competes and wins. He gets a trip to New York where he's enabled to take dance classes at Broadway Dance Center, Alvin Ailey and other dance schools. A dream comes true for this 18 year old who wasn't familiar with contemporary dance. His solo was a 5 minute dance routine on I wanna melt with U, a funky pop track from The Artist Formerly Known As Prince and consisted of a mix of vogue, jazz, funk, hiphop, ballet, African dance,... and was the start of Cherkaoui's personal movement language. It was built on his own choices, free of any interference, free of any opinions or schooling. At that time Cherkaoui felt he was putting together what he liked in dance; the jury saw emerge something unique and personal. (Eastman)

Later, while studying at P.A.R.T.S, he encountered the dance of William Forsythe, Pina Bausch and Trisha Brown, took classes in theatre, sociology, dance history and learnt De Keersmaeker's Rosas repertoire. Parallel with his contemporary training, he worked with hip hop companies and modern jazz groups in Belgium. Cherkaoui ended his education at P.A.R.T.S prematurely after only one year of study to join Les Ballets C. de la B. as a performer in Platel's work *Iets op Bach* (1997–1998), a successful dance theatre production with a worldwide tour, further instilling a sense of global citizenship in Cherkaoui.

In 1999, Cherkaoui danced and choreographed *Anonymous Society*, which was co-written with Andrew Wale and Perrin Manzer Allen. The musical won the 'Fringe First Award' and the 'Total Theatre Award' in Edinburgh, while in London it received the 'Barclay Theatre Award' in 2000. While he was touring *Iets op Bach*, Cherkaoui created a work for the Flemish Polydans company, entitled *Afwezen (fatalidad)*, his first avenue into choreographing for dancers. Soon afterwards he joined Les Ballets C. de la B. as a choreographer, presenting work that seemed influenced by Platel's dance theatre. *Rien de Rien*, his first choreography as a member of the artistic core of Les Ballets C. de la B., toured throughout Europe, winning the 'Special Prize' in Belgrade at the BITEF Festival in 2001. The production was created in collaboration with cellist Roel Dieltiens. One of the dancers and singers in the productions, the French-Belgian Jalet, stimulated Cherkaoui's interest in vocal music and would become one of Cherkaoui's key long-term collaborators. In cooperation with Nienke Reehorst, Cherkaoui spent a year working with mentally disabled actors, which resulted in the performance *Ook* (2002) by the theatre company Theater Stap in Turnhout, Belgium. Reehorst, too, continued to work with Cherkaoui as choreography assistant, particularly for works for large groups of performers.

In 2002, he took part in the 'Vif du Sujet' at the Festival d'Avignon with the solo *It* (2002), directed by Wim Vandekeybus. In collaboration with Jalet, Luc Dunberry and Juan Kruz Diaz de Garaio Esnaola (dancers/singers with Sasha Waltz), the work *d'avant* (2002) was created for the Schaubühne am Lehniner Platz in Berlin, Germany. This work can be considered a precursor to *Foi*, in the sense that the performers explore songs from the tenth to thirteenth century. Cherkaoui won the Nijinsky Award for 'Emerging Choreographer' at the Monaco Dance Forum in 2002. In 2003, he created *Foi* with Les Ballets C. de la B. in collaboration with Dirk Snellings and Capilla Flamenca, and this production won the prize of 'Best Choreography' at the First International Movimentos Dance Awards in 2004.

Having outlined important developments in Cherkaoui's early life and the beginnings of his choreographic career, it becomes clear that, despite his unusual entry via television and variety shows into the dance world, his work—created from the start in a transnational collaborative network—began to receive recognition at home and abroad. To continue this brief biography of Cherkaoui and the overview of his career, in 2004 the Festival d'Avignon invited him to create *Tempus Fugit*, which was co-produced by Pina Bausch's Tanztheater Wuppertal. The main musical collaborator for this work was Najib Cherradi and the ensemble Weshm. At the end of 2004, Cherkaoui premiered *In Memoriam*, commissioned by the prestigious Les Ballets de Monte Carlo, featuring the renowned Flemish ballerina Bernice Coppieters, under the artistic leadership of Jean-Christophe Maillot. The work is an ode to the departed, inspired by the people in Cherkaoui's family who passed away, and marked the beginning of a period of collaboration with the Corsican *a capella* ensemble A Filetta, led by Jean-Claude Acquaviva.

Early 2005 saw Cherkaoui commissioned by the Grand Théâtre de Genève; the resulting *Loin* explored the themes of travelling, distance and culture shock. In July, Cherkaoui partnered up with director Andrew Wale again for the musical *Some Girls Are Bigger Than Others*, based on the music of Morrissey and The Smiths. Cherkaoui also resumed his co-creation with Khan that summer and premiered *zero degrees* in London in July 2005, only a few days after the London 07/07 bombings. In August 2005, Cherkaoui and Nicolas Vladyslav created a duet in collaboration with Dieltiens, entitled *Corpus Bach*. In 2006, Cherkaoui and Jalet co-choreographed *Aleko* for the Tokyo International Arts Festival. Later that year, *Mea Culpa* followed as Cherkaoui's second creation for Les Ballets de Monte Carlo, collaborating with Delmas for the set design and Karl Lagerfeld for the costumes. Another commission followed in 2006, for the Cullberg Ballet led by Johannes Inger; this work was entitled *End*. In 2006, Cherkaoui also became associate artist at Het Toneelhuis, the municipal theatre company of Antwerp.

2007 was a year of creative energy for Cherkaoui, as it started with the premiere of *La Zon-Mai* and a duet for Iris Bouche and Damien Fournier, *Intermezzo*, created in his new role as associate artist at Het Toneelhuis. He was also commissioned to choreograph *L'Homme de Bois* for the Royal Danish Ballet to the music of Igor Stravinsky's *Pulcinella*. However, the year was dominated by the creation and premiere of *Myth*, Cherkaoui's first major work for Het Toneelhuis and a collaboration with Patrizia Bovi's Ensemble Micrologus and set designer Wim Van De Capelle. In the latter half of 2007, Cherkaoui struck up a partnership with La Monnaie/De Munt opera in Brussels, for which he choreographed *Apocrifu*, with musical accompaniment by the Corsican *a capella* ensemble A Filetta.

In 2008, Cherkaoui created *Origine* for Het Toneelhuis, a work for four dancers representing the extremities of the compass: north, south, east and west. In the spring, he premiered the large-scale Sadler's Wells production, *Sutra*, featuring monks of the Shaolin Temple in China, a second set design by Antony Gormley and music score by Szymon Brzóska. The year 2009 started with *49-Jae*, a solo for the Korean dancer Nam Jin Kim and *The House of Sleeping Beauties* for Het Toneelhuis and La Monnaie/De Munt. He also choreographed sequences for Flemish theatre group Olympique Dramatique's musical *Adam's Appels*. He was commissioned to create *Orbo Novo* for Cedar Lake Contemporary Ballet in New York, as well as marked the centenary of the Ballets Russes at

Sadler's Wells with his duet *Faun* for Daisy Phillips and James O'Hara. Towards the end of 2009, Cherkaoui co-choreographed the duet *Dunas* for himself and flamenco dancer María Pagés. The end of Cherkaoui's prolific first choreographic decade was marked by the founding of his own dance company, Eastman, in January 2010, which then presented *Babel*^(words) in April as a first work in co-production with La Monnaie/De Munt and co-choreographed with Jalet.

Babel^(words) is the third and final part of two distinct trilogies. On the one hand, Cherkaoui had framed the succession of his works *Foi, Myth* and *Babel*^(words) as a trilogy exploring the depths of humanity and culture. These three works stage a series of interactions between a set of worldly protagonist actors—notably Christine Leboutte, Ulrika Kinn Svensson and Darryl E. Woods—and a chorus of otherworldly dancers representing angels, shadows and national communities, respectively. *Foi, Myth* and *Babel*^(words) were performed consecutively as a trilogy at the Grande Halle de La Villette in Paris in June and July 2010. On the other hand, *Babel*^(words) is also the third work created in collaboration with the visual artist Gormley, after *zero degrees* and *Sutra*. The designs for these three works progressively widen the way the body is framed: in *zero degrees*, latex dummies cast off the performers' bodies are the result of a close enveloping, while in *Sutra* a set of wooden boxes provide personal hiding space and shelter, and finally in *Babel*^(words) oversized, open, metallic cuboid frames continually transform the performance space and direct the spectator's gaze to the dancing bodies' activities within. The works of these two trilogies culminating in *Babel*^(words) were Cherkaoui's main artistic focus in the 2000–2010 period and, together with *Rien de Rien* and *Apocrifu*, will be the key works discussed in this book.

The end of the first decade of the new millennium brought the launch of Cherkaoui's dance company, Eastman, wholly dedicated to the production of his choreographies, of which *TeZukA* (2011), *Puz/zle* (2012) and *Fractus V* (2015) are perhaps the most notable. However, the ever-prolific choreographer also continues to maintain artistic partnerships with the world's most renowned institutions and artists beyond this company alone. For Sadler's Wells, he created *m¡longa* (2013), based on both an ethnographic exploration of tango and a collaboration with Argentinian artists. A collaborative creative endeavour with Chinese dance artist and choreographer Yabin Wang resulted in the group work 生长*genesis* (2013).

Furthermore, he has continued to pursue creative projects within popular culture, for example his choreographing for music videos by Icelandic band Sigur Rós, his work on Cirque du Soleil's *Michael Jackson ONE* (2013), and his choreographic collaboration with Beyoncé for her 2017 Grammy Awards performance and music video for the single 'APESHIT', which she released with JAY-Z, set in the corridors of the Louvre. A partnership started between Cherkaoui and theatre and film director Joe Wright, first for the feature film *Anna Karenina* (2012), starring Keira Knightley and Jude Law, and then for the Young Vic production *A Season in the Congo* (2013) with actor Chiwetel Ejiofor. Cherkaoui also took on the movement direction of Lyndsey Turner's *Hamlet* (2015) at the Barbican, with Benedict Cumberbatch in the starring role. New are Cherkaoui's contributions to the development of opera: in the period 2010–2013, he worked with director Guy Cassiers on Richard Wagner's *Der Ring des Nibelungen*, choreographing *Das Rheingold* and *Siegfried*. For the commemoration of the start of the Great War, Cherkaoui choreographed and directed the opera *Shell Shock* (2014) at De Munt/La Monnaie in Brussels. In 2018, Cherkaoui also turned his hand to musicals again, choreographing Diablo Cody's rock music *Jagged Little Pill*, inspired by Alanis Morisette's album of the same name, for the American Repertory Theater. Meanwhile, choreographic commissions for ballet companies have continued to form a key pillar of Cherkaoui's oeuvre, most notably *Boléro* (2013), co-choreographed with Jalet and in collaboration with Marina Abramović for the Ballet de l'Opéra National de Paris and *Memento Mori* for Les Ballets de Monte Carlo.

When the Royal Ballet Flanders was looking for a new artistic director following the departure of Assis Carreiro in 2014, the Board of Governors' attention soon turned to the world-renowned choreographer who was virtually living on their doorstep in Antwerp and approached Cherkaoui. He took up the position from February 2015 and has put his extensive expertise in working with ballet dancers to use in his own creations for the company, for example *Fall* (2015) and *Requiem* (2017). Moreover, Cherkaoui's insights and worldwide reputation and connections are also deployed in securing choreographic commissions and repertoire works from renowned artists for the company, for example works by Martha Graham, Pina Bausch, Yuri Grigorovich, Ohad Naharin, Crystal Pite, Meryl Tankard, Edouard Lock and Annabelle Lopez Ochoa. As such, he takes a transcultural dramaturgical approach to shaping the ballet company's season of works with which spectators are invited to engage. However, Cherkaoui's extensive experience with opera must be of considerable interest to the now merged ballet and opera organisation. A first venture into close ballet and opera collaboration in 2018 was *Pelléas et Mélisande*, conceived and designed by Abramović and co-directed and co-choreographed by Cherkaoui and Jalet.

In my overview of Cherkaoui's activities since 2010, I have been unable to list and mention all facets of his creative portfolio. I hope, however, that I have been able to convey a sense of his ongoing commitment to collaboration and interdisciplinary and cross-cultural exchange, as well as the impact this mid-career choreographer has been able to have on audiences around the world. His rise from autodidact teenaged dancer, discovered by Platel in 1995 to Artistic Director of Royal Ballet Flanders in 2015 has been phenomenal and testament to his astute artistic vision and relentless, but intelligent work over the years.

KALEIDOSCOPIC IDENTITY AND AESTHETICS

The Belgian political imagery of rainbow coalitions and mosaic structures offers potential to be expanded to conceptions of identity and Cherkaoui's choreographic aesthetic. With regard to the concept of identity, Cherkaoui repeatedly indicates that he has been influenced by Amin Maalouf's *In the Name of Identity: Violence and the Need to Belong*. In this book, Maalouf puts forward the notion of composite identity or the idea that a person's individual identity is a 'special case', 'complex, unique and irreplaceable' (Maalouf 20) and made up of several links to different groups of people. 'Every one of my allegiances links me to a large number of people. But the more ties I have the rarer and more particular my own identity becomes' (Maalouf 18). Cherkaoui states:

> I am half-Flemish, half-Moroccan, blond, I have a tattoo on my back, I am homosexual… I am the sum of multiple identities. When one of our identities is put in danger, it becomes more important than the others. When I hear homophobic statements, I am homosexual. When I hear racist statements, I am Arabic. However, I constantly try to remember that I also consist of other, equally important identities. (qtd. in Hervé)

'L' homme kaléidoscope'—or kaleidoscopic man—is the term used to reflect on Cherkaoui's conception of identity by visual artist

Justin Morin, who published a brief publication of conversations with Cherkaoui about his philosophical stance and cultural concerns (Morin 8). The metaphor of the kaleidoscope implies an ever-shifting movement of small fragments of coloured glass, suggesting that Cherkaoui acknowledges that identity is not fixed but constantly reoriented. It also means that, for Cherkaoui, national identity is only one aspect of identity and he would be cautious of letting it overpower the other dimensions of his identity. In Maalouf's writing on identity as composite and characterised by multiplicity, Cherkaoui found affirmation of his kaleidoscopic approach to identity as fragmented, ever-shifting and constantly realigned and reoriented. For Cherkaoui, national identity is but one aspect of identity and he is cautious of allowing it to overpower the other dimensions of identity.

In Cherkaoui's key large group works from the previous decade, *Rien de Rien, Foi, Tempus Fugit*, and *Myth*, the kaleidoscope is a useful image to describe the mise-en-scène, in which—at certain times—multiple little scenes happen simultaneously and centrifugally, away from centre stage. Kaleidoscopic configuration also recurs in the split screens and ever-shifting images of *La Zon-Mai*.

The chapters that follow will grapple with the kaleidoscopic structures and multiple layers of meaning of which Cherkaoui's works consist. The kaleidoscope aesthetic has a profound impact on the experience of the spectator in processing the simultaneous and ever-shifting mise-en-scène. The rest of the book will evaluate the impact that Cherkaoui's work makes on cultural attitudes towards the nation, language, history and religion through close analysis of his key works. Each chapter will present an example of what this extended, continuous dramaturgy of the spectator might look like. Chapter 2 focuses on *Rien de Rien* as a choreographic and dramaturgic response to the Belgian political context of instability and impasse, tainted by the rise of the Flemish populist radical right, from Cherkaoui's personal subjectivity. The work is used as a case study to discuss Cherkaoui's mise-en-scène, choreographic preoccupations and the implications of the complex dramaturgy for the spectator. In Chapter 3, the concept of transculturalism is introduced through analysis of *zero degrees*. A particular emphasis is placed on the significance of storytelling and song in Cherkaoui's work, and the chapter theorises the travel story as a site in which cultural friction comes to the fore. *Sutra* is also discussed in Chapter 3 as a work in which Cherkaoui explores the limits of transculturalism. Chapter 4 foregrounds

Cherkaoui's choreographic explorations of religion in *Foi* and *Apocrifu*. The chapter explores the notion of the transreligious in relation to these two works, entertaining the possibility that the context of the rise of religious fundamentalism may be resisted and countered through an emphasis on how different religions are linked and continuously influencing and transforming each other. Chapters 5 and 6 both take as their central focus the large-scale and multi-layered work *Myth*. Chapter 5 is concerned with Cherkaoui's dramaturgical strategy of including multiple languages in his work without translation; the chapter interrogates the consequences of this heteroglossic dramaturgy of non-translation on the spectator, drawing on postcolonial critiques of translation which are given prominence in recent translation studies. Still in relation to *Myth*, Chapter 6 evaluates how Cherkaoui—with the aid of Jungian psychoanalytical notions—repositions religion as a kind of myth. The analysis of *Myth* explores the potential of the tools of Jungian dream analysis for the dramaturgical labour in which the spectator engages in response to the complex theatrical images Cherkaoui presents. Chapter 7 begins to prepare key conclusions about this first decade of Cherkaoui's choreographic oeuvre through analysis of *Babel*^(words)^, in terms of how the choreographers' thinking about culture, nation and language has developed under the influence of critical geopolitics. The final Chapter 8 reflects on the ways in which the choreographic themes, micro-dramaturgical strategies and macro-dramaturgical concerns that emerge from Cherkaoui's work intersect with one another and what this analysis can tell us about engaged spectatorship.

Finally, I want to end this introductory chapter with a brief note on the importance of descriptive analysis for this research. Throughout the book, I delve in and out of a descriptive mode of writing in my engagement with the selected works by Cherkaoui. Here, the writing employs Janet Adshead's seminal *Dance Analysis* model, which is based on breaking the dance down into its minimal components (performers, movements, visual elements, aural elements) and separating out the labour of the analyst into different stages: describing the components, discerning the form of the dance, interpretation and evaluation. While acknowledging the immediate limitations of this model, I will make a case for the benefits of engaging in extended description of the work as a whole. Here, the main purpose of extended description is to convey a sense of the overall multiplicity and complexity of the work. Moreover, the act of translating spectatorial experiences into written words allows writer and reader to develop a shared sense of the mise-en-scène of the work, an understanding of how the choreographer puts images and sounds together, even though it is understood that the written account is always already subjective and an incomplete, imperfect record. However, my choice for employing Adshead's *Dance Analysis* is also at the same time a point of departure from this model and other semiotic performance analysis models (Foster; Pavis). The premise of the book is that Cherkaoui's work seems to demand an analytical engagement from the scholar that goes far beyond these performance analysis models, a custom-made analytical approach that will enable the scholar to respond actively to the deep cultural questions Cherkaoui raises in his work about identity, culture, nation, religion and language. From my descriptive analyses of the works emerge my research questions: What does the labour that Cherkaoui invites me as a spectator to engage in entail? How will I respond to the big cultural questions Cherkaoui poses in his work? Will I, as a spectator and researcher, and others around me transform the ways we think about life, about the world?

NOTE

1. In 2004, the VB party was convicted for inciting racial hatred and changed its name from Vlaams Blok (Flemish Block) to Vlaams Belang (Flemish Interest).

BIBLIOGRAPHY

Adshead, Janet. *Dance Analysis: Theory and Practice*. London: Dance Books, 1988. Print.

Bossuyt, Reinout & De Lobel, Peter. 'Maak uw Eigen Coalitie'. *De Standaard Online*. 2011. Web. Accessed: 2 August 2011. <http://www.standaard.be/extra/verkiezingen/2010/coalitiekiezer>.

Bousetta, Hassan & Jacobs, Dirk. 'Multiculturalism, Citizenship and Islam in Problematic Encounters in Belgium'. *Multiculturalism, Muslims and Citizenship: A European Approach*. Ed. Modood, Tariq et al. Oxon: Routledge, 2006. 23–36. Print.

Brah, Avtar. *Cartographies of Diaspora: Contesting Identities*. Gender, Racism, Ethnicity Series. Oxon and New York: Routledge, 1996. Print.

Cherkaoui, Sidi Larbi. *Curriculum Vitae*. 1999. Unpublished Manuscript.

———. 'Eén achternaam, veel toekomst'. *MO Magazine*. 2014. Web. Accessed: 13 August 2017. <http://www.mo.be/artikel/een-achternaam-veel-toekomst>.

Cherkaoui, Sidi Larbi & Delmas, Gilles. *Zon-Mai: Parcours Nomades.* Arles: Actes Sud, 2007. Print.

Clifford, James. 'Diasporas'. *Cultural Anthropology.* 9.3. (1994): 302–338. Print.

Deschouwer, Kris. 'And the Peace Goes On? Consociational Democracy and Belgian Politics in the Twenty-First Century'. *West European Politics.* 29.5. (2006): 895–911. Print.

De Standaard. 'Fotospecial: De crisis gezien door kinderogen'. 2011. Web. Accessed: 15 June 2011. <http://www.standaard.be/artikel/detail.aspx?artikelid=DMF20110611_024>.

Doran, Meredith. 'Negotiating Between *Bourge* and *Racaille*: Verlan as Youth Identity Practice in Suburban Paris'. *Negotiation of Identities in Multilingual Contexts.* Ed. Pavlenko, Anna & Blackledge, Adrian. Clevedon: Multilingual Matters, 2004. 93–124. Print.

Eastman. 'Project/Best Belgian Dancesolo'. 2018. Web. Accessed: 24 August 2018. <http://www.east-man.be/en/14/56/>.

Foster, Susan L. *Reading Dancing: Bodies and Subjects in Contemporary American Dance.* Berkeley: University of California Press, 1986. Print.

George, Rosemary Marangoly. *The Politics of Home: Postcolonial Relocations and Twentieth-Century Fiction.* Berkeley: University of California Press, 1999. Print.

Gilroy, Paul. *The Black Atlantic: Modernity and Double Consciousness.* London: Verso. 1993. Print.

Hervé. 'Sidi Larbi Cherkaoui sur le Pont'. *Têtu.* July/August 2004.

Jackson, Merilyn. 'Review: Zon-Mai'. *Philly Stage.* 2011. Web. Accessed: 19 August 2017. <http://www.philly.com/philly/blogs/phillystage/Review-Zon-Mai.html#fBYZ8qWsM4OzoYD6.99>.

Lefkowitz, Natalie. *Talking Backwards, Looking Forwards: The French Language Game Verlan.* Tuebingen: Gunter Narr Verlag, 1991. Print.

Maalouf, Amin. *In the Name of Identity: Violence and the Need to Belong.* New York: Random House, 2000. Print.

Mnookin, Robert & Verbeke, Alain. 'Persistent Nonviolent Conflict with No Reconciliation: The Flemish and Walloons in Belgium'. *Law and Contemporary Problems.* 72:151. (2009): 151–186. Web. Accessed: 18 July 2011. <http://www.law.duke.edu/journals/lcp>.

Morin, Justin. *Sidi Larbi Cherkaoui: Pèlerinage Sur Soi.* Arles: Actes Sud, 2006. Print.

Mudde, Cas. *The Ideology of the Extreme Right.* Manchester: Manchester University Press, 2000. Print.

———. *Populist Radical Right Parties in Europe.* Cambridge: Cambridge University Press, 2007. Print.

Pavis, Patrice. (trans. David Williams) *Analyzing Performance: Theater, Dance, and Film.* Ann Arbor: University of Michigan Press, 2003. Print.

Peeters, Patrick. 'Multinational Federations: Reflections on the Belgian Federal State'. *Multinational Federations*. Ed. Burgess, Michael & Pinder, John. Oxon: Routledge, 2007. 31–49. Print.

Renard, Han & De Ceulaer, Joël. 'De 10 machtigste en invloedrijkste allochtone landgenoten'. *Knack*. 2014. Web. Accessed: 17 July 2017. <http://www.knack.be/nieuws/mensen/de-10-machtigste-en-invloedrijkste-allochtone-landgenoten/article-normal-125747.html>.

Ryan, Stephen. 'Nationalism and Ethnic Conflict'. *Issues in World Politics*. Ed. White, Brian et al. 3rd Ed. Basingstoke: Palgrave Macmillan, 2005. 137–154. Print.

Seymour, Michel. *The Fate of the Nation State*. Montreal: McGill-Queen's University Press, 2004. Print.

Stevens, Mary. 'Le CNHI on Tour: la Zon-Mai and the Visual Identity'. 2007. Web. Accessed: 17 August 2017. <http://marysresearchblog.wordpress.com/2007/03/21/the-cnhi-on-tour-la-zon-mai-and-the-visual-identity/>.

Sturtewagen, Bart. 'Weg uit Logica van Winaars en Verliezers'. *De Standaard*. July 2011. Print.

Tierney, Stephen. *Accommodating Cultural Diversity*. Farnham: Ashgate, 2007. Print.

Vincendeau, Ginette. *La Haine*. I.B. Tauris, 2005. Print.

Multimedia Sources

Bye Bye Belgium. RTBF. 2006. Online Video. Accessed: 21 December 2012. <http://www.youtube.com/watch?v=O1OcwJPK3Vo>.

La Zon-Mai. Created by Sidi Larbi Cherkaoui and Gilles Delmas. Lardux Films. 2007. Web. Accessed: 18 July 2014. <http://www.zon-mai.com/accueil_fr>.

Interview

Cherkaoui, Sidi Larbi. Interview with author 4. Antwerp, June 2007.

CHAPTER 2

Rien de Rien—Dramaturgy Inviting an Engaged Spectatorship

Premiered in 2000, *Rien de Rien* was Cherkaoui's choreographic debut under the auspices of Les Ballets C. de la B., following Cherkaoui's participation as a dancer in Alain Platel's *Iets Op Bach* (1999). *Rien de Rien*'s extended European tour and its numerous choreographic awards foregrounded the choreographer in the international dance field, while framing him as an outsider to the established Flemish dance scene. A young, 'allochthonous' (immigrant), and inexperienced choreographer, who lacked formal dance training, Platel's protégé caught the spectators' and critics' eye. This chapter offers a choreographic and dramaturgical analysis of *Rien de Rien*, in which the work is read as a disarming critique of the Flemish populist radical right, nationalism and xenophobia, made from the viewpoint of Cherkaoui's plural cultural identity. The work is a helpful tool to introduce Cherkaoui's oeuvre in the 2000–2010 decade and the choreographic themes and dramaturgical strategies he pursues in this time, as well as the influences of key collaborators that have shaped his vision and approach. In this chapter, I identify five key choreographic themes and six dramaturgical strategies that will form the focus of this book.

The key choreographic themes introduced in *Rien de Rien* and developed by Cherkaoui in later works are: gestural hand movements and choreographed storytelling; the citation of popular and folk dance practices; circular movements akin to calligraphy; manipulation, power play and a literal objectification of dancing bodies; and extreme virtuosity, contortionism and inversion. Many dramaturgical strategies developed in

© The Author(s) 2019
L. Uytterhoeven, *Sidi Larbi Cherkaoui*, New World Choreographies,
https://doi.org/10.1007/978-3-030-27816-8_2

Cherkaoui's later work are introduced in *Rien de Rien*: a creative exploration of postcolonial and 'Other' subjectivity; the privileging of orally
transmitted songs and stories; heteroglossia and non-translation of foreign languages; choreographed iconography of a religious nature to be
excavated; and a complex mise-en-scène characterised by simultaneity.
This chapter explores the connection between the dramaturgical complexity of *Rien de Rien* and the political complexity of the Belgian state,
discussed in the introductory Chapter 1. The complexity of Belgium's
political structures may have inadvertently played a role in resisting the
rise of the populist Flemish radical right, which was the surrounding
context in which Cherkaoui began to create around the turn of the millennium. His experience as a young person of Moroccan heritage, growing up in this political climate, may have influenced him in embracing
complexity as a deliberate dramaturgical strategy in his choreographic
work. The choreographic and dramaturgical elements listed above are
indexical of wider cultural issues Cherkaoui addresses in his body of
works in the 2000–2010 period, which are explored further in subsequent chapters.

The musical landscape is an indication of *Rien de Rien*'s eclecticism
and a direct result of the work's diverse cast. Cherkaoui is joined as a
performer by the French-Belgian Damien Jalet, who went on to become
Cherkaoui's longstanding artistic collaborator throughout the decade, fuelling the choreographic oeuvre with traditional songs from the
Mediterranean region, extreme physical risk-taking, absurd humour and
political astuteness. The Jamaican-born singer and dancer Angélique
Willkie also contributes to the range of songs in the work through her
rendition of Edith Piaf's 'Rien de Rien', Sam Brown's 'Stop' and a
traditional African song. The final musical partner is the renowned
Belgian cellist Roel Dieltiens, who brings contemporary scores by Luc
Van Hove, Sofia Gubaidulina, György Ligeti and Zoltán Kodály to the
work's aural landscape. Dieltiens sits holding his cello on a raised platform stage left and remains detached from the proceedings on the
wooden dance floor, bordered with Moroccan rugs, commenting only
with his music. Jalet, Willkie and Cherkaoui are joined by three more
dancers on stage: Cherkaoui's ballet teacher Marie-Louise Wilderijkx, the
teenaged Laura Neyskens and the Slovenian dancer Jurij Konjar. Several
scenes in which two or more performers recount travel stories in various languages in unison, complete with synchronous gestures, are particularly memorable. Other suggestive theatrical imagery in *Rien de Rien*

includes Konjar clambering on Arabic, Qur'anic calligraphy on the wall and the Francophone Jalet spray-painting the plea 'Flemish, please' onto Cherkaoui's back while Willkie sings Piaf's 'Rien de Rien'. The work is laced with irony and absurdity, which continually undermines the serious tone of any scene in a way that is perhaps characteristic of a pre-9/11 mode of making dance theatre.

This chapter also historically locates Cherkaoui's practice within both Flemish and Anglophone discourses on new dramaturgies around the turn of the millennium, which are concerned with decentring dramaturgy away from the single figure of the professional dramaturg. I argue that due to the particular factors that characterise the dramaturgical collaboration at the heart of *Rien de Rien*, this work and the dramaturgical strategies advanced within it helped to shape the discourse on and practices of new dramaturgy. For *Rien de Rien* Cherkaoui worked with dramaturg Hildegard De Vuyst, who had long been connected to Les Ballets C. de la B. and Platel. The time of creation coincided with her article 'A Dramaturgy of Shortcoming' in the Flemish theatre journal *Etcetera*, in which she reflects on the power imbalances between emerging artists and the dramaturgs who are thrust upon them by producers to fill a perceived lack of ability. This initial dramaturgical collaboration between Cherkaoui and De Vuyst provided a blueprint for Cherkaoui's later works: an experiential and spectatorial dramaturgy that jolts the spectator into a re-evaluation of established cultural identities and values.

Historical Development of New Dramaturgies and Discourses in Flanders

Cherkaoui's work both emerged from and influenced the Flemish discourse on new, non-text-based dramaturgies since the 1990s (Van Kerkhoven, De Vuyst, Van Imschoot), which in turn has been influential on recent European and North-American conceptions of, and approaches to, dance dramaturgy (Turner & Behrndt; Hansen & Callison; *Contemporary Theatre Review*; *Performance Research*). An exploration of the collaborative, dramaturgical processes shaping Cherkaoui's choreographies in the early 2000s allows readers to refine their understanding of how new approaches to negotiating the issues of power, agency and labour in transcultural dance dramaturgical practices emerged at the turn of the millennium. Along with that of Platel,

Anne Teresa De Keersmaeker and William Forsythe, Cherkaoui's work was part of a wider trend in dance dramaturgical collaborations that urged scholars to refocus the discourses on dramaturgy, away from defining the role of the professional dramaturg as a solitary figure responsible for dramaturgy.

Defining dramaturgy itself remains difficult as there is a multitude of complex practices to which the term applies. The pioneer Flemish dance dramaturg Marianne Van Kerkhoven conceived of dramaturgy as a twofold function. On the one hand, it refers to both 'the internal structure of a work' and to the dialogic and 'collaborative process of putting the work together' (Van Kerkoven qtd. in Turner & Behrndt 17). On the other hand, it also implies an analytical function in the interplay between the work and the spectator, moving 'beyond the idea that the drama contains a simple set of signifiers for us to decode' (Van Kerkhoven qtd. in Turner & Behrndt 18). In this book, it will be argued that certain choices Cherkaoui makes in the composition of his works deliberately aim to complicate signification. Hence, the two functions are intertwined and inseparable, like the two sides of a coin.

The concept of 'new dramaturgy' emerged from a wave[1] of significant collaborations between choreographers and dramaturgs within the Flemish contemporary dance scene since the 1980s (Van Imschoot 'Anxious dramaturgy' 58). The artistic collaborations were paralleled by an invigorated theoretical discourse in Flemish theatre journals, such as *Theaterschrift* and *Etcetera*, about the nature of this new kind of dramaturgical work. A key figure in this discourse is Van Kerkhoven, who worked with, among others, De Keersmaeker at the Kaaitheater in Brussels in the 1980s. Van Kerkhoven's seminal text 'Looking Without Pencil in Hand' which is published in four languages,[2] proposes her professional experiences as a model for dramaturgical working methods and is generally regarded as the starting point of the discourse. She wrote at a time when the description, and pinning down, of the dramaturg's activities would enable further discussion. It triggered a chain of critical responses, among others from dramaturgs De Vuyst and Myriam Van Imschoot, and therefore created a fertile climate for consideration of the new developments with an increasingly international outlook.

Yet most discourses on dramaturgy did not take into account the full concept of dramaturgy as laid out in the above tentative definition of the term in its totality and mainly focused on the collaborative relationship between an artist and a professional dramaturg or an analysis of the role of dramaturgy in the creative process. My experiences with Cherkaoui's creative practice and choreographic work, however, led me to question whether more emphasis was required on the broader concept of dramaturgy, as something which is not limited to the professional activity of a dramaturg, nor to the creative process alone. Dramaturgical practice is not, and need not, always be tied to collaboration with a named dramaturg. Although Cherkaoui employs a dramaturg to work on certain larger productions, for example De Vuyst, Guy Cools or Lou Cope, on other occasions he works without one, and this does not imply that dramaturgical activity, therefore, does not take place. The early Flemish discourse on new dramaturgies expressed anxieties about the dramaturg as a figure of power and proposed an extended conception of the term dramaturgy to include a range of people, not only the dramaturg. In the special issue of *Women & Performance*, Van Imschoot demonstrated the possibility of political agency stemming from the dramaturg's invisibility, stating that this 'shapeshifter who is hard to locate […] can operate more freely in the wings' (Van Imschoot 'Anxious Dramaturgy' 57). Paradoxically, it was noted, however, that the figure of the dramaturg had recently been subject to a heightened interest from scholars and had therefore become more visible.[3] Van Imschoot located the dramaturg's agency in 'a process of legitimization, validation and control […] well beyond the close collaboration with the artist' (Van Imschoot 'Anxious Dramaturgy' 57). However, the sense of agency was extended by another, perhaps more severe, power relationship, which located the dramaturg as part of a complex economic system of intermediary functions designed to interface between the artist and the audience. This system ultimately 'discourage[d] direct artistic participation', because by '"voice"[-ing] artistic concerns' dramaturgs 'silence[d] those for whom they are speaking' at the same time (Van Imschoot 'Anxious Dramaturgy' 62). Artists like Cherkaoui at the start of his career—young, 'allochthonous', and inexperienced as a choreographer—were perceived to be in need of somebody to help them articulate their artistic vision more clearly and hence allocated a dramaturg.

However, to avoid silencing those for whom dramaturgs speak, Van Imschoot suggested a reformulation towards 'more dramaturgical contexts' in which 'an ongoing dialogue about the work' could be held between multiple partners 'without the mediating filter of "the" dramaturg' (Van Imschoot 'Anxious Dramaturgy' 63). Van Imschoot confided that in these kinds of conversational contexts she dreaded being labelled the 'dramaturg'. This statement indicates a struggle with the negative connotations of the term and a reluctance to identify with the concept of the dramaturg as a figure of authority. Her conclusive statement to the text was strong and decided: 'you do not need a dramaturg to achieve the dramaturgical' (Van Imschoot 'Anxious Dramaturgy' 65). Van Kerkhoven similarly argued for the role of 'interlocutor'[4], not necessarily the dramaturg, but someone with whom the artist could discuss his/her work (Van Kerkhoven 'Grote Dramaturgie' 67). This shift in perception of the dramaturg addressed a perceived problem with the power-relationships between the artist and the dramaturg and proposed a move beyond confining dramaturgical responsibility to a single authorial figure.

This need to differentiate between dramaturgy and the dramaturg was shared as a main concern in the early European discourses on new dramaturgies. Apart from the creation of dramaturgical contexts, another alternative option to diminish the role of the dramaturg was the idea of a shared dramaturgical responsibility with the performers. Not only was the performer key in 'creat[ing] a bridge between choreographer and the public' in order for 'the dramaturgical vision of the choreographer [to] becom[e] clear' but performers have also evolved into making or being asked to make both choreographic and dramaturgical decisions themselves as a result of new collaborative choreographic methods at the turn of the millennium (deLahunta 'Dance Dramaturgy' 23). As a result, the 'intellectual responsibility of the piece is shared with the whole group', instead of being 'singled out into [the] position and [...] function' of the dramaturg (deLahunta 'Dance Dramaturgy' 24). Van Imschoot's notion of 'a collective and active responsibility for all the components' was embedded in Cherkaoui's creative processes I observed ('Anxious Dramaturgy' 65).

Through the substitution with a dramaturgical context, a definite impulse to lift the figure of the dramaturg out of dramaturgy could be discerned in these historic discourses. This correction to the perception of dramaturgy could be seen as a response to the political implications of the 'division of labor' in choreographer/dramaturg collaboration, a topic Van Imschoot was particularly concerned with (Van Imschoot 'Anxious Dramaturgy' 65). Some of the main activities of the dramaturg involve words (talking, writing). Van Imschoot voiced the concern other dramaturgs share with her that the allocation of language and discourse to the realm of the dramaturg may indicate in some instances that the dramaturg was compensating for a lack or perceived lack of knowledge or intellectual capacity.

The necessity of the figure of the dramaturg was first questioned in a polemic in Flemish theatre journals *De Witte Raaf* and *De Vlaamse Gids*, respectively, by Meuleman and Melens (De Vuyst 'Dramaturgie'). In her response, De Vuyst concluded that in the framework of old-fashioned theatre practice in which the polemic originally took place, dramaturgy indeed fulfilled the role of 'legitimisation and didactics'[5] of dance and theatre (De Vuyst 'Dramaturgie' 66). In this process, 'the dramaturg is the embodiment of a shortcoming',[6] a perceived lack of structural integration or historiographic design (De Vuyst 'Dramaturgie' 66). In essence, she criticised the employment of the dramaturg with the aim of compensating for a perceived lack of capability within the artist. In line with the general views, she suggested different strategies to support artists in a broader dramaturgical context. The performance maker and theorist Bojana Cvejić later agreed with De Vuyst and Van Imschoot that 'it's important that a dramaturg doesn't enter the process because the process is in need of a dramaturg' (Cvejić 48). She suggested, along with philosopher Jacques Rancière, that the emancipation-ignorance paradigm might be useful for conceiving of the relationship between the choreographer and the dramaturg. Trusting that spectators are emancipated, active and capable of fulfilling their responsibilities in the signification process, Cvejić proposed that the dramaturg and choreographer 'establish a relationship of equals' characterised by ignorance about the work they are about to create and engage with (Cvejić 44).

The reluctance to use the term dramaturg and the attempt to relocate dramaturgical activity into alternative realms could be read as an impulsive reaction to the sudden realisation that the dramaturg was situated on the exploitative side of the power equation. Brizzell and Lepecki confirmed the existence of 'a diatribe against dramaturgs (but *never* against dramaturgy)' (Brizzell & Lepecki 15). The historic discourse on dramaturgy had surpassed its initial functions of self-definition and self-legitimisation. At first glance, by reflecting on their professional practice, many dramaturgs merely suggested preferable ways to regard dramaturgical activity. However, by raising awareness of issues such as the political implications of the division of labour within choreographer/dramaturg collaboration, the discourse also developed a function of self-regulation. The creation of dramaturgical contexts and the concept of dramaturgically engaged spectatorship are suggested in this book as alternatives to the problematic notion of the figure of the dramaturg as a single person of authority. With regard to Cherkaoui's

work, dramaturgical strategies are collaboratively shaped and dramaturgical responsibility is shared by the choreographer(s), dramaturgs, choreographic assistants, performers, musical directors, visual designers and the
technical team. What follows in this chapter is a detailed analysis of these
collaboratively shaped choreographic themes and dramaturgical strategies
in *Rien de Rien*, which ultimately push spectators towards a dramaturgical engagement with the work and its political implications.

CHOREOGRAPHIC THEME 1: GESTURAL HAND MOVEMENTS AND CHOREOGRAPHED STORYTELLING

At the start of *Rien de Rien*, two women, Willkie and Neyskens, enter
the stage space via a door in the wooden wall at the back. They walk
in unison along the edges of the dance floor, approaching a couple of
microphones on stands downstage. They take a breath together and
begin to tell a story about travelling in—presumably—Africa, a camel
journey and reaching a village, where the narrator, presumably Willkie, is
welcomed by the local people. Their voices tell the story in unison. Their
gestures are identical and perfectly synchronised. A subtle shift of weight,
sinking into the hip. A flick of the wrist. A tilt of the head. Eyes lift up,
as if remembering the experience or looking for the right words. A shrug
of the shoulders. They scratch behind their ear and uncomfortably look
down at the floor. The scratching turns into hair twiddling. Emphatic
nods. Meanwhile, three male dancers lift their chests off the floor and
hop and slide sideways across the floor. My attention as a spectator is
torn between watching three men, Cherkaoui, Jalet and Konjar, who are
performing intricate floor movements spinning on their heads, and listening to the women's story. I cannot do justice to both at the same
time. Then, I notice that the men's movement patterns rhythmically
align themselves to the patterns in the women's speech. For a moment,
I enjoy the musicality of the narration and seeing how the floor choreography visualises the breath and timbre of the voices.

The women's gestures become more animated when they talk about
the killing of a goat, which is done in celebration of Willkie's arrival as
a guest in the village. The story mentions two little boys who play with
the animal's head, while the blood is still leaking out of it. The boys
kick it, pick it up by the ears, spin it around and put it on a stick. The
women physicalise these actions. To hilarious effect, it is revealed that

the storyteller is vegetarian. While the story addresses the notion that in the West people do not really have to deal with where meat comes from, the three men embark upon a new movement pattern: facing the back wall, which has Arabic writing across it, they stand, kneel and bow down, to then stand up again and repeat the whole pattern numerous times. This coincides with the women narrating about having respect for the animal, in the sense that an animal is only killed when it is truly necessary and that, because of that animal, people can live and survive. Juxtaposing this part of the story with an image of Islamic prayer, Cherkaoui evokes a thought of the ritual slaughter of livestock, which some members of the Muslim community in Belgium tended to do in their gardens to celebrate the end of Ramadan. These actions by their Muslim neighbours made some Flemish people uneasy. Cherkaoui thus alludes to cultural tensions between Flemish people and Muslim immigrants. More generally, food and religious customs are both very closely connected to culture. When encountering others, either as a result of travelling, as is the case for Willkie, or of migration, these cultural aspects tend to reveal cultural friction early on. Hence, they form the part of Cherkaoui's exploration of cross-cultural experiences in this work.

Later in *Rien de Rien*, Willkie tells a story about a man in robes, who is resting his hand on her leg during a journey in a van. In a culture in which touching or even making eye contact with women is forbidden, the man knows he is not supposed to be doing this. Cherkaoui visualises elements of the story about the hand with gestures involving his hands on his own body: he places his hand down on the floor; he traces his fingers over his stomach; and he grabs on to his forearm, while his breathing accelerates and becomes shallower, shoulders slightly tense. He rests his hand on the top of his thigh and looks down at it, as if it is not his own. Different aspects of sexuality come into play: this story and Cherkaoui's visualisation of it introduces the notion of masturbation and the defying of religious dictates around sex. Willkie says that she did not mind the hand being on her thigh, but wishes she had found the courage to look around at him. As several hours pass, she says she had grown accustomed to the hand being there. This story is a second fragment of Willkie's larger travel story, which is woven through the work as a dramaturgical red thread. Both the fragmentation of the story and the duplicating of the storyteller's voice and body language by another dancer work to heighten the spectator's perception as an invitation to engage more deeply and more creatively with the work's dramaturgy.

Further choreographic and gestural elements are added to extend the resonance of the storytelling. Cherkaoui amplifies Willkie's gestures in a tense, exaggerated manner with a locking and popping movement quality. Willkie mentions a goat hanging off the side of the van, echoing the goat from the opening story. She talks about a snake flying through the air. He falls forward, onto his shoulder, head turned sideways. Jalet launches himself across and around the space, jumping and turning energetically like a coiled spring being released, or perhaps that snake Willkie was talking about. Cherkaoui makes a peace sign. He wants to move his foot forward, but it is stuck to the ground. He releases it quickly and his foot hits the back of his head, repeatedly. The floor seems magnetic, and he needs to use his hands to manoeuvre his legs across the floor. His hand covers his eyes, his ears, his mouth and then his crotch. He brings his hand up to hold his throat. He slaps himself across the cheeks and thumps the palm of his hand against his forehead. Clasped hands move towards his mouth as if holding a microphone. He gestures as if pointing a gun at someone, then points it against his own temple. He extends his fingers, palm down against temple, as if saluting. Then, he pulls his hand across his brow as if peering into the distance. He holds his hand up to the side, palm forward, as if greeting someone, then extends his arm to become a Hitler salute. He pulls back his elbow and closes his fist, as if he is about to punch someone. He moves from a peace sign to sticking up his middle finger. He extends his index finger and pinky as in a heavy metal gesture. All the while, the other, free hand intervenes to adjust the gesticulating hand to the next position. This choreographic sequence of random yet recognisable hand gestures shows how small subtleties of non-verbal communication can have a big impact on meaning; yet also draws attention to the arbitrariness of the semiotic sign and the potential margin of error in any communication. The manipulation of one hand by the other indicates Cherkaoui's disrupted or warped sense of agency in his subjectivity as an 'allochthonous' young man.

In her analysis of the role of the hand in Cherkaoui's choreography, the dance anthropologist Krystel Khoury reads its significance in the following way: 'Being the ultimate mode of communication, the hand is at times a way of narrating, a way of manipulating and of expressing. Playing the role of the trigger of the movement, it is above all that by which one creates the dance. In short, it allows Sidi Larbi Cherkaoui to leave his fingerprint on his creations. As he says: "What's great about hands is that there are all these possibilities. There are so many things one can do with one's fingers. Expression is the greatest with one's hands. It's also the part of the body that one uses the most during the day and that with which one identifies the best. [...] In fact, someone's identity is that person's hand."' (Khoury 26) The choreographic strategy of unison storytelling recurs throughout Cherkaoui's oeuvre in different guises, notably in *zero degrees* (co-choreographed with Akram Khan). The implications of Cherkaoui's emphasis on travel stories for his development of transcultural dramaturgies is analysed further in this chapter. Other works, such as *Foi*, *Apocrifu* and *Babel*$^{(words)}$ (co-choreographed with Jalet), too, include elements of rehearsed storytelling, whether duplicated in other bodies or not.

Choreographic Theme 2: The Citation of Popular and Folk Dance Practices

In the middle of *Rien de Rien*, Konjar and Wilderijkx perform a tango duet, footwork only, accompanied by the cello. She gazes the young man in the eye with desire, and he looks back nervously and with a little trepidation. Meanwhile, Neyskens brushes her meter-long hair, which comes down to her waist and then re-braids it. By the end of the tango, Neyskens has finished braiding her hair and it has been transformed into a weapon, a whip of some sort. Neyskens and Konjar embark on a different partnered social dance: the lambada. The cello plays pizzicato and then the sound fades away, so that most of this duet is performed without music. All we hear is the tapping of sneakers on the floor. There are intricate patterns in the duet, arms weaving in and out of each other, performed at great speed. Konjar jerks Neyskens around quite a bit. She wears a red bikini bra and a red mini skirt that swings up when her hips rotate, revealing big white underwear. The big underwear adds not only a comical visual effect; it also represents Neyskens's childhood and signals that she has not quite reached an adult level of sexual maturity. In the middle of the Lambada duet, Konjar takes off his shirt, and this is greeted by Neyskens's ecstatic wide-open mouth. Willkie bursts out in laughter at the absurd scene of youthful courtship. By having the tango duet with Wilderijkx followed by the Lambada duet with Neyskens, Konjar is depicted as a man who could pursue sexual relationships with women both older and younger than him.

The duet finishes with acrobatic lifts, during which he tosses Neyskens over his shoulder and across his hips. Eventually, he throws her into the wings, while she lets out a panicky, piercing squeal. Konjar remains unattached to either woman, old or young, beyond the ephemeral moment of the dance they shared.

Throughout his oeuvre between 2000 and 2010, Cherkaoui continues to mine popular and folk dance as a source of dance movement in his works, for example Slovakian folk dance and tap dance in *Myth* (2007), flamenco in *Dunas* (2009, co-choreographed with María Pagés), Kuchipudi in *Play* (2010, co-choreographed with Shantala Shivalingappa), Bollywood dancing in *Foi* (2003) and break dancing in *Babel^(words)* (2010, co-choreographed with Jalet). His citation of popular and folk dance practices offers an alternative to the Western, 'high art' movement idioms of ballet and modern or postmodern dance that serves to call into question dance theatre's choreographic aesthetic. It enables the performers in the work to introduce their cultural specificity in the same way that their speaking of different languages does, which Cherkaoui already explores in *Rien de Rien* and which will be the focus of discussion in Chapter 5. In this sense, Cherkaoui's citation of popular and folk dance practices is connected to the dramaturgical strategy of exploring postcolonial or Other subjectivity, which will be explored later in this chapter. However, in *Rien de Rien*, by using Konjar and the Lambada and Wilderijkx's experience of the tango as his starting points, Cherkaoui immediately posits dance and movement practices as globalised and not inherently tied to local cultures of origin. He, therefore, undermines any quest for authenticity, recognising that dance practices—and people—travel from place to place and their meanings shift accordingly.

CHOREOGRAPHIC THEME 3: CIRCULAR BODILY MOVEMENTS AKIN TO CALLIGRAPHY

After Willkie has finished telling the story about the man in robes placing his hand on her thigh in the back of a van, she utters the phrase 'There is nothing more seductive than the forbidden', which anecdotally I discovered is what the Arabic calligraphy in bas-relief on the back wall translates as. Cherkaoui, Jalet, Neyskens and Konjar execute a fluid arm choreography in unison, while Willkie continues the story. Standing in one place, feet firmly anchored, both hands move up to the shoulders, elbows jutting out. Then, the forearms and hands gracefully unfold and drop down again. While the upper body is twisted to one side, one wrist initiates a diagonal movement across the torso, which has twisted round to the other side in the meantime. Sequentially, the left and right arms lift, fold, rotate and sink, cascading up and down the torso, which twists from side to side. Hands move up to the side of the face and back down again. Fingers linked, the hands frame the face with angular wrists. Cherkaoui's fingers reach to the side, while the other dancers continue to repeat the fluid arm choreography. He lets his fingers lead the rest of the body into turns, into a kneeling position and back up. He lifts and extends his leg up to his hands, which are held high above his head. His hands reach backwards down to the floor, and Cherkaoui's body follows through into a slow and measured backflip. His two index fingers meet in a cross shape, which morphs into a peace sign. Cherkoui mimics hanging himself. He falls back into the unison arm movement with the other dancers. It strikes me how similar the lines traced by the hands through the space are to the Arabic calligraphy on the back wall.

These ever-looping arm movements recur as a motif in many of Cherkaoui's works, notably in those in which he works with ballet companies. For example, in *In Memoriam* (2004) for Les Ballets de Monte Carlo and in *Fall* (2015) for the Royal Ballet Flanders, the dancers perform continuous circular arm movements like those in *Rien de Rien* while performing *bourrées en pointe*, largely remaining stationary. Cherkaoui's circular arm movements are akin to the hand twirls and air screw motions found in waacking, although Cherkaoui often tends to connect both hands together at the fingertips or wrists. As such, the movements resemble a figure of eight or an infinity symbol that is enlarged, diminished, twisted and spun out into endless three-dimensional variations of the shape.

A similar approach exists with the whole dancing body, which in Cherkaoui's choreographies often spins, twists, circles and turns into and out of the floor in fluid, endless sequences. Often these circular dance phrases are performed by solo male dancers accompanied by *a capella* singing, for example, Nicolas Vladyslav in *Foi* (2003), James O'Hara in *Myth* (2007) and Dimitri Jourde in *Apocrifu* (2007). The combination of agility, strength and control in their dancing is almost otherworldly and superhuman.

CHOREOGRAPHIC THEME 4: MANIPULATION, POWER PLAY AND A LITERAL OBJECTIFICATION OF DANCING BODIES

After the opening story told by Willkie and Neyskens, Cherkaoui suddenly launches into a quick dance that visualises the exact structure of the Belgian composer's Luc Van Hove's irregular cello score. The dance is cartoon-like and comical, as Cherkaoui bumps into Willkie, prompting her to join in. There are traces of popular dance movements, such as the framing of the face found in vogueing. The structure of both music and dance is very unpredictable. There are none of the usual run-ups or preparations for jumps and turns as is common in codified dance techniques, such as ballet. The dancers move as if they are animated puppets or avatars stuck in a computer game. In this disorderly scene, Cherkaoui and Willkie, as the two dancers who are the most Other—an 'allochthonous' young man and a black woman—are represented as being entirely acted upon with the frantic, unpredictable music dictating their every movement. Initially, it is they who are depicted as having no agency, tugged and shoved around the space by invisible forces at an extraordinary pace. Eventually, a number of white dancers also join in, suggesting that everyone's identities and actions are shaped by discourse; no one is an entirely free agent. Jalet bumps into Willkie like a bulldozer, oblivious to his actions, his white masculinity trampling over her black female body, which is inconveniently in the way of his path. At the end, Cherkaoui falls flat on his front, his face turned to the side, utterly exhausted.

Towards the end of *Rien de Rien*, in a compelling duet, Cherkaoui's rigid body is balanced on Konjar's thigh. A now completely naked Willkie sings a traditional song. Konjar swings Cherkaoui onto his shoulder. He balances him upright, with one arm around his neck and holding onto a raised leg. He balances a rigid Cherkaoui onto his back. Cherkaoui leans into Konjar's chest. He hangs upside down in front of Konjar's body, his lower leg hooked over Konjar's shoulder. Konjar flips him around so that their fronts are now touching each other, Cherkaoui still upside down. He slides Cherkaoui down until his head is on the floor. Konjar spins him slowly around, walking around him. The whole-body manipulation continues, as Cherkaoui seems completely powerless to direct his movements, yet great strength is required for him to hold his body stiff and stable in these precarious positions. Cherkaoui balances on Konjar's thigh and leans back, Konjar holding on to him by his shoulder. He holds Cherkaoui upside down, legs in the air. Konjar kneels and Cherkaoui arches back across his thigh. Konjar crosses Cherkaoui's arms and holds him in his arms like a Pietà figure, but after only a few seconds Cherkaoui's head slips through and he dangles upside down. Cherkaoui's body is depicted entirely like a lifeless puppet, an object to be manipulated. In this scene, Cherkaoui has choreographed his own self-objectification, his ultimate lack or loss of agency. It could be argued that he is depicting the objectification of immigrants or those perceived as 'allochthonous' in the context of the Flemish populist radical right. Konjar places Cherkaoui standing on the floor, but Cherkaoui's eyes are downcast, his head tilting down. Konjar lifts Cherkaoui's chin and buttons up his shirt (Fig. 2.1).

From the way in which the work has been constructed dramaturgically, the link between the choreographed loss of agency and Cherkaoui's subjectivity as the son of a Moroccan immigrant growing up in late-twentieth century Flanders is a key realisation that draws the whole work together in the mind of the spectator. With his own

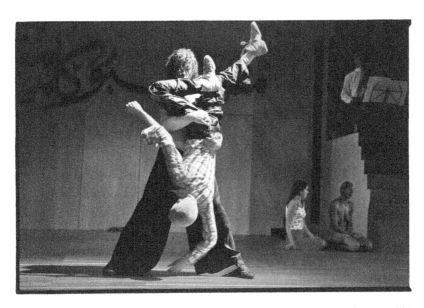

Fig. 2.1   Jurij Konjar, Sidi Larbi Cherkaoui, Laura Neyskens, Angélique Willkie and Roel Doeltiens in *Rien de Rien* (Photo by Chris Van der Burght)

self-objectification, from loss of agency with his movements being dictated by the music or his body parts being manipulated by his own hand to becoming a puppet to be handled by another performer, Cherkaoui visualises how the Flemish populist radical right objectifies 'allochthonous' people. It becomes possible to read in Cherkaoui's duet with Konjar, a whole-body manipulation of increasing invasiveness, a critique on the everyday violence done onto those rendered powerless by populist discourses.

The notion of the puppet is one that Cherkaoui revisits in different contexts in future works, notably the latex dummies designed by Antony Gormley in *zero degrees* (2005) and the wooden Bunraku-inspired puppet in *Apocrifu* (2007). Beyond working with physical puppets, Cherkaoui often choreographs the interactions of manipulation between people. For example, in *Foi* and *Myth*, the protagonists are manipulated by angels and shadows, respectively, who lightly but decidedly coerce the protagonists into their daily actions while hovering in their personal space. At other times, the interactions turn more violent, for example the shadow fights influenced by martial arts in *zero degrees* and *Myth*. *Babel*$^{(words)}$ sees quite a few hustle and bustle scenes, in which the performers struggle with each other over space and territory. Here, too, the fights are with an invisible power at times, for example Helder Seabra's solo in the aluminium cuboid frame, which reminisces the notion of a dancer's movements being driven by external, invisible forces, like in the cartoonesque scene from *Rien de Rien* described previously.

CHOREOGRAPHIC THEME 5: EXTREME VIRTUOSITY, CONTORTIONISM AND INVERSION

After finishing the long sequence of hand gestures, Cherkaoui commences jogging on the spot again, his feet dragging but not travelling forwards. He looks over his shoulder, as if someone is chasing him and begins to run full out. He drops onto his knees and his head bumps onto the ground. He gets back up, changes direction and falls again, this time coinciding with the other two men kneeling down into a prayer action. While Jalet and Konjar's praying action is smooth and measured, Cherkaoui's head—although in the same position as the praying men—bumps onto the ground with an audible thud. This lack of control also points to Cherkaoui's unease with having to operate within the constraints of religion. The two men increase the intensity of their energetic choreography moving across the stage, speeding up towards exhaustion. Cherkaoui places a pointed gun finger against his temple, mimics shooting himself and stumbles towards the back wall, until his chest is pressed up against it, head turned to the side, arms splayed. This is the same position as when he fell on the floor, only now vertical up against the wall. He drags his body sideways, almost unnoticeable, but leaves a trace of blood smeared on the wall.

Towards the end of the work, Konjar suddenly gets up, lifts Cherkaoui upside down and carries him to the back, where he leans Cherkaoui against the wall on his head, arms by his side. It is that same posture Cherkaoui was in before, when he fell onto his front and when he ran into the wall; only this time, he is upside down. He stays like that for several minutes. I imagine that it must be extremely difficult to stay in that position, that it must be uncomfortable, painful even, to only carry the weight of your body on your head for that long. Not until the end of the work do I hear a thud coming from the darkness and wonder if it is Cherkaoui who has fallen.

In future works, Cherkaoui continues to deliberately exploit inversion, a basic tenet of yoga, as a choreographic strategy. He has indicated in a conversation with me in 2014 that he is interested in the change of perspective on the world that comes from being upside down. Added to this is the extreme strength and control of the body, which Cherkaoui pursues in virtuoso movement material in, for example, *zero degrees*, where it is combined with extreme hypermobility. Another example is a handstand in *Foi*, held by Vladyslav for a length of time while the other performers around him shake and make the ground rumble with their stamping feet to evoke an earthquake.

With regard to choreographic themes 3, 4 and 5, the notion of affect seems pertinent. One of the objects of the emerging discipline of affect studies is to analyse how affect is elicited by text or works: 'affect denotes sensations, intensities, valences, attunements, dissonances, and interior movements shaped by pressures, energies, and affiliations embedded within or made part of diverse forms of embodied human life' (Wehrs & Blake 3). The notion of affect has gained significant traction in dance studies as well, for its complex relationship to the body of both doers and watchers of dance. Dance and theatre scholar Timmy De Laet cites recent advances in affect theory (Gregg & Seigworth) in defining affect as the 'visceral forces beneath, alongside, or generally other than conscious knowing' (34). He draws on the philosopher Brian Massumi in explaining that affect is of an 'irreducibly bodily and autonomic nature' (34). De Laet further summarises that affect 'provides a name for those supposedly unmediated sensations that elude conscious registering' (34). Many of Cherkaoui's choreographic approaches work to elicit affect from spectators. The never-ending circular movement sequences, the manipulations of and sometimes violence done to literally objectified dancing bodies, and the inversion and contortionism leading to extremely virtuosic choreographic material all work to implicate spectators on an affective level, impossible to register consciously. The closest I come to it in my own experience is recognising I feel my skin tingle, feel warm and energised inside, or sometimes feel deeply uncomfortable watching the choreography, to the point of feeling pain sensations. It will be illustrated at various parts in the book how this is connected to the wider dramaturgically engaged spectatorship developed in response to Cherkaoui's work.

I will now begin to identify six key dramaturgical strategies that are introduced in *Rien de Rien* and further developed by Cherkaoui in subsequent works. These dramaturgical strategies begin to form the analytical skeleton for the rest of the book, as their significance is considered more deeply in the remaining chapters.

DRAMATURGICAL STRATEGY 1: A CREATIVE EXPLORATION OF POSTCOLONIAL AND 'OTHER' SUBJECTIVITY

In heterogeneous works such as *Rien de Rien* and the other 2000–2010 works that are the focus of this book, Cherkaoui actively shaped his works through a careful curation of which performers and collaborators he worked with. A diverse range of performers, in terms of nationality, ethnicity, 'mixedness', age, languages spoken and artistic practices, was often the starting point. Through the collaborative creative process, these cultural elements and the particular experiences and stories of the performers would become the dramaturgical building blocks in the works. In this endeavour, Cherkaoui grew more deliberate throughout the decade in working with artists who would challenge Western dance theatre aesthetics and Eurocentric and hegemonic world views. Difference and 'otherness' also include disability in this context, notably the casting of performers with Down's Syndrome: Marc Wagemans in both *Foi* and *Myth*, and Ann Dockx in *Myth*.

This emphasis on difference and diversity as a starting point and creative driving force forms part of Cherkaoui's life project of endeavouring to understand the experiences of others around him and to strive towards better communication and cooperation with others. The remaining chapters in this book, through their focus on language, religion, culture and national identity, analyse the ways in which Cherkaoui invites spectators to join him in this quest through various dramaturgical strategies leading to an engaged spectatorship.

DRAMATURGICAL STRATEGY 2: THE PRIVILEGING OF ORALLY TRANSMITTED SONGS AND STORIES

As a key collaborator in *Rien de Rien*, Jalet brought considerable expertise in traditional Mediterranean song under the influence of ethnomusicologist Giovanna Marini. This becomes present in the work through the Italian popular religious hymn 'Stabat Mater Dolorosa', a hymn that was suppressed by the Church as heretic in the Council of Trent during the Counter-Reformation. Jalet and Cherkaoui harmonise bare-chested, one standing behind the other, evoking Christian iconography through four-handed gesturing. This interest in orally transmitted song would stay with Cherkaoui throughout the decade that follows and beyond (Fig. 2.2).

Apart from orally transmitted stories, this chapter has already touched upon some of the stories told in *Rien de Rien*, in the context of the choreographed storytelling. Later in the work, Willkie and Konjar tell another story in unison, about a foreign marriage ritual, where a whole village looks in on the bride-to-be in a hut, saying 'I've never experienced anything like this. My god, what are they doing? [...] I mean, for her, even with whatever apprehension she must feel, it's completely normal'. The story is located at the tension between feminism and cultural relativism, unsure about whether to be shocked at the lack of the woman's rights and the perceived sexual violence done to her, and the ethnographic fascination with the rituals of the Other. It echoes debates held in Flemish media about the wearing of headscarves by Muslim women and the practice of arranged marriages. The story goes mute, while Willkie continues to gesture and mouth the words, indicating that this has been only a fragment of the story. It becomes possible to connect this story to the one told at the start of the work, about the killing of

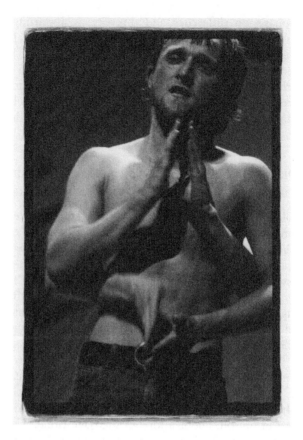

Fig. 2.2 Damien Jalet and Sidi Larbi Cherkaoui in *Rien de Rien* (Photo by Chris Van der Burght)

the goat, as perhaps having happened during those same travels. Hence, disparate layers of meanings begin to accumulate; yet, spectators must actively remember and link them together in order to see the larger picture.

Towards the end of *Rien de Rien*, Neyskens and Jalet enter through the door, moving in unison. They casually walk up to the microphone downstage and begin audibly breathing and chewing into the microphone. Jalet tells a story in French about being invited to share a meal in a foreign country, and Neyskens performs the accompanying gestures with him in unison. He talks about there being a fire in front of a hut, and the leader of the village having many wives. He is offered a few sheets of some sort of paste in a little bowl, just like the villagers are holding. While they eat it, unfortunately one of his travel companions asks what it is they are eating. They discover that the food is prepared by being chewed and spat out. So, Jalet says, everyone had the same thought: Should they take it out of their mouth or not? He starts to blush. He says that he did not want to put the food on the muddy ground.

Stories and orally transmitted songs continue to be a significant feature of Cherkaoui's oeuvre from 2000 to 2010 and beyond.[7] Orality is a key focus in the work of literary theory scholar Walter Ong. He connects the shift in Western culture from orality to literacy to rising linearity in thought, visualist tendencies and individuality. Cherkaoui expresses a distrust of the written word—particularly the Word of God—in several of his works, notably *Foi* and *Apocrifu*; hence, the privileging of stories and orally transmitted songs in his works may be a deliberate attempt to preserve non-written forms of remembering and passing on knowledge—much like dance is an oral and embodied cultural practice— and the community aspects associated with orality.

DRAMATURGICAL STRATEGY 3: SELF-REFLEXIVE, DANCE HISTORICAL REFERENCES

Quite early on in *Rien de Rien*, Wilderijkx enters the stage space, wearing black flowing trousers, high heels and carrying white voile wings. She sweeps through the space in elegant whirls, reminiscent of Loie Fuller's dances, which are etched into my memory not only from photographs and film fragments that remain, but also from the art nouveau sculpture by François-Raoul Larche and drawings by Henri Toulouse-Lautrec inspired by this modern dance pioneer. Konjar whistles the tune of 'The Dying Swan' from *The Carnival of Animals* (1905) by Camille Saint-Saëns, the dance which made Anna Pavlova famous. Wilderijkx is thus framed as the embodied voice of dance history and tradition in the work. She is also Cherkaoui's ballet teacher. He did not take up ballet training until he was a young adult, perhaps searching for a counterbalance to the autodidacticism that characterises his path into professional dance through popular show dance and hip hop. Wilderijkx nearly mows down the other performers with her wings; they duck out of the way. Still, on balance, this dominance of dance traditions does not take hold in the work, and Wilderijkx remains somewhat of an outsider in this work, perhaps not as fully immersed in the creative methodologies Cherkaoui employs as the other performers.

Later, Neyskens stands behind her and wraps her long, braided hair around Wilderijkx's neck, pulling her off the stage, evoking the death of another key dance historical figure, Isadora Duncan, who was strangled when her scarf got entangled in the wheels of a convertible car. With this cartoon-like gesture, Neyskens yanking Wilderijkx off stage also sets up the two women as antagonists. The then 16-year old Neyskens seems to be trying to claim her rightful spot in the sphere of femininity, while Wilderijkx appears to resent Neyskens's youthful girlishness. Considering the work's apparent emphasis on femininity and female experience, Wilderijkx's choice of dance historical heroines begins to make sense: Pavlova, Fuller and Duncan are all early modern dance figures that speak to the imagination.

Later on in the work, Wilderijkx gives a cringe-worthy impression of dance history from a Western, ballet-centric perspective. She begins by doing an exaggerated walk with knees bent up high and elbows and wrists flexed. The walk might be read as vaguely African and alludes to what might be offered in some dance history books as 'primitive' dance, taken to stand for the early beginnings of dance. In her seminal 1970 essay 'An Anthropologist Looks at Ballet as a Form of Ethnic Dance', Joann Kealiinohomoku debunks the assumption that it may be possible to derive what primeval dance looked like by examining the dances of primitive people in the now; yet, Wilderijkx reinstates this imperialist approach to dance history in her solo. Wilderijkx goes on to evoke Egyptian hieroglyphs by moving in parallel on a straight line, her hands and arms flexed on that same line. Considering a postcolonial context, the dance is just 'all wrong' in the connections that it draws. She then performs what looks like Balkan-style folk dancing, in which dancers hold on to each other's shoulders in a circle and click their heels together. Next, an impression of the Romantic ballet is given through soft arm gestures in a sylph-like manner. She swiftly moves on to the virtuosity of classical ballet, by executing an *entrechat quatre* jump in fifth position, and an *arabesque* lifting the leg to a 90-degree angle. The dance suggests a teleological progression through time towards the high-point of classical ballet, the style of dance with which Wilderijkx most closely identifies. The second half of the dance shows a decline, in which the ideals of classical ballet are abandoned or wilfully rejected. The verticality of the body is shifted to a more diagonal and grounded exploration of the body's kinesphere as happens in modern dance techniques, such as those devised by Martha Graham, José Limón or Merce Cunningham. She places her two hands around her neck in a strangling gesture and rounds her back as in a Graham-style contraction. Only, by this point, I have noticed that Wilderijkx only creates the shapes of these Other dances—non-ballet dances—in a static way, moving from one position to the next, but without really connecting the movements in an embodied way. It reminds me of the way in which national dances were embedded in Romantic and classical ballets of the nineteenth century, for example, Spanish, Indian or Slavic dances, to give an exotic flavour of local colour: a quickly recognisable gesture or posture is imitated and linked together in a balletic movement vocabulary. Wilderijkx loosely kicks her foot to the side and casually lifts the opposite shoulder, in a jazzy way. She walks forward framing her face with her hands as in vogueing. She finally performs a fragment of a pivoting phrase, which I recognise from De Keersmaeker's *Fase* (1982), a key reference point in Belgian contemporary dance history. When this whistle-stop tour of 'dance history around the world' is completed, she repeats it, only slightly faster. This nugget of choreography is well-contained and included in the work almost as a citation. While Wilderijkx performs it with the most serious, deadpan expression, it is surrounded by little absurd, cartoonesque and slapstick elements, eventually leading me to get over my initial anger and imagine its ironic inclusion as a possibility. Whereas the work up to that point had mostly featured popular dances, choreographed gestures, or movement material arising from improvisation, it typifies Cherkaoui to seek out unusual ways like these, in collaboration with the performers and the movement vocabularies with which they feel comfortable, to engage in dialogue with the codified dance world through the creative process.

A decade later, Cherkaoui and Jalet go on to include further self-reflexive dance historical references in *Babel(words)*, suggesting a recurring interest in questioning their own place with mainstream dance histories. In *Rien de Rien*, Cherkaoui opts to keep the imperialist, 'wrong' dance historical reference firmly separate from the rest of the work, indicating that he as a postcolonial figure is critical of this approach. Furthermore, as an autodidact he does not seem to wholly identify with the way dance historical meanings have been created within institutions

to the exclusion of Other dance and movement practices that do no fit
within the established Western concert dance aesthetic.

DRAMATURGICAL STRATEGY 4: HETEROGLOSSIA
AND NON-TRANSLATION OF FOREIGN LANGUAGES

After her Loie Fuller-inspired whirling dance, Wilderijkx tells a story in
French about being taken to Antwerp station in cold weather, being well
dressed in the family heirloom fur coat, collar and hat. She and her travel
companions are made to board an airplane without knowing the details
of the journey in a time when things had to be mysterious, then make
an emergency landing. The airplane's doors open to let in a minus 30
degrees cold. The story is told by Wilderijkx, Willkie and Cherkaoui, in
canon, each starting a few seconds after one another. The canon pattern
makes it difficult to follow and understand the story; instead, I am only
able to pick up fragments here and there and am forced to piece together
meaning from those. They later fall back into unison and then go back
to speaking in canon. They talk about not speaking the language, not
knowing what is happening nor why, and experiencing a sense of confusion. This confusion is mirrored in the staggering of voices in the canon
storytelling, making the spectator work extra hard to derive meaning
from the scene.

Konjar and Willkie immediately launch into a story about cultural
biases in English. The switch from French to English emphasises the
stark differences between the two languages, the people who speak them
and the attitudes, sensibilities, affectations and gestures that accompany
them. Those in the audience who were lucky enough to understand both
languages would have included many Belgians. However, the advantages
afforded by multilingualism exceed the functional, the ability to directly
trade and work with people outside your country without the need for
translation. Cherkaoui is framing multilingualism as an ability to understand and culturally connect with Others, one of life's gifts of growing
up in Belgium. This celebration of Belgian multilingualism is in stark
contrast to the Flemish nationalist populist radical right, which insists on
language purity. The abrupt changes between languages again jolt the
spectator into active listening.

After Neyskens and Konjar's lambada duet, Wilderijkx walks up
to the microphone, grimaces and exclaims a few sentences in Russian:

'You probably haven't got children, do you? You don't have children. In the army, there is everything and we haven't got anything'. Because I don't speak Russian, I was unable understand this text while watching the performance. The only link I could imagine was that, perhaps, Wilderijkx had spent some time in Russia as a ballerina, enabling her to pick up the language. It was not until later, when I showed a video to a friend, that I could understand these few sentences. Then, they echoed the kind of thing that is often said to childless people, especially women: that until or unless they have children, they cannot fully know what love is. Drawing attention to something like this highlights another facet of female experience.

At the very end of *Rien de Rien*, Konjar begins to tell a final story, in Slovenian. All I can deduce is that it talks about the mountains, the Alps, because he mimics the action of downhill skiing. Willkie joins in with the talking and the accompanying gestures, in unison. Struggling to understand the content, I am drawn to the musicality of the storytelling again. Neyskens, Wilderijkx and Jalet come over and join in the gesturing. Then, the story dies down.

Heteroglossia and non-translation are a key dramaturgical strategy in the majority of Cherkaoui's works, particularly *Foi*, *Myth* and *Babel*$^{(words)}$. Chapter 5 will approach this issue in more depth, by exploring the implications of existing postcolonial critiques of translation. In terms of engaged spectatorship, spectators inevitably have to work harder to surpass their cultural bias and engage in cross-cultural dialogue with others or further research to begin to understand certain dramaturgical layers of the work, or else face being excluded by the foreign languages spoken or sung.

DRAMATURGICAL STRATEGY 5: CHOREOGRAPHED ICONOGRAPHY OF A RELIGIOUS NATURE TO BE EXCAVATED

Immediately after Wilderijkx's brief utterance about not having children in Russian, Cherkaoui stands behind Jalet, both men shirt-less. Jalet begins to sing the Latin song 'Stabat Mater Dolorosa', taking long pauses in between certain syllables. It is a Christian hymn evoking the Virgin Mary standing next to Jesus on the cross, weeping. In the light of the Russian text that immediately preceded it, this image—a juxtaposition of the loss of a child with the notion of childlessness—becomes all the more poignant. Cherkaoui gently joins in, singing in harmony. The two men evoke Christian iconography through four-handed gestures, raising arms, joining hands, touching Jalet's head and chest. They bring their fists up to Jalet's forehead, suggesting a thorn crown. Jalet brings his index finger to Cherkaoui's palm, alluding to the stigmata. Although the imagery is religious, homoerotic tension is building through the two semi-nude men's closeness and gentle touching. The song is very moving, with emotions building as the *a capella* voices fill the space with more and more force. The other dancers also join in the harmonies. The two men point with their index finger up and down on the final notes of certain verses, visualising the piercing high and low notes on which they end. These pointing gestures become larger towards the climactic ending of the song. The final gesture sees Cherkaoui holding his forearm in front of Jalet's neck and cutting his own arm with a knife, which could signify both murder and self-harm.

Later, Neyskens enters wearing a giant hooped white wedding dress. She rides a unicycle and falls off after only a few seconds. She twists from side to side, so that the hoop continues to spin around her. She performs some ballet *changement* jumps and curtseys. She balances the back of the hoop on top of her heard, creating a giant halo. She brings the two palms of her hands together in front of her chest, a Christian praying gesture. She makes coquettish gestures and eye movements. She picks up her unicycle, moves towards the door and turns around to open the door, revealing the bright red miniskirt she was wearing earlier. By combining a few simple actions with a gratuitous prop and excessive costume, a completely absurd theatrical image is created that gently pokes fun at Catholic sanctimony that permeates Flemish folklore. Meanwhile, Konjar has started to clamber on the Arabic writing on the back wall, an act that might be considered as sacrilegious.

Later, the back wall becomes significant again as a backdrop against which choreographic imagery is played out. Willkie has lost the Tina Turner wig, revealing blonde curls, and begins to stammer Edith Piaf's 'Rien de Rien', already out of breath from dancing frantically, which she continues to do. She has taken off her dress and is dancing and singing topless wearing just black shorts. While the crouching and semi-nude Willkie sings 'Rien de Rien' out-of-breath, Jalet looks at her in disdain, hands resting on his hips. He looks at the wall and back at her. He walks towards the wall, takes a can of spray paint out of his pocket and shakes it. He sprays the slogan 'Vlaams aub!' ('Flemish please!') onto the wall, probably referring to the French lyrics of the song Willkie is singing. This is ironic, as Jalet is Francophone (Belgian-French). The exclamation mark is placed neatly onto the motionless Cherkaoui's back, the dot onto his bottom. With this single action—a plea for language purity, punctuated onto the body of an 'allochthonous' young man—the work calls into question the populist radical right's conflation of the Flemish independence agenda with xenophobia and Islamophobia.

The rest of this book, but particularly Chapter 6, is concerned on the excavation of the rich and complex theatrical imagery presented by Cherkaoui and his collaborators, particularly religious iconography in *Myth*. It is impossible to take these images at surface value if spectators are concerned with deriving meaning from the works. Each work contains several visual conundrums that invite further reflection, dialogue and research, and hence, spectators are invited to revisit the imagery over the days, month, years even that follow and deepen their engagement with the works. In the process, by opening themselves up to the cultural practices of Others, they may begin to question their own cultural identity and accompanying world view.

DRAMATURGICAL STRATEGY 6: COMPLEX MISE-EN-SCÈNE, CHARACTERISED BY SIMULTANEITY

Rien de Rien repeatedly reinforces the diversity of this community of seven performers: the different languages they speak, different generations and ethnicities they belong to, different nationalities, different dance vocabularies, different musical tastes and different dramaturgical agendas they carry. The fragmented stories keep spectators guessing as to their specific context or relevance. Furthermore, the tango, performed to only very sparse notes on the cello, offers a pause for the spectator to let the dramaturgical layers on femininity sink in: there are three women in this work—a teenager, a middle-aged woman and a slightly older one. They connect with each other in different ways: through imitation, through looking and at times through struggle, competing for male attention. Sandwiched in between these elements of female experience is a story about the bride-to-be, a story which alludes to the larger question of women's rights in other cultures. The work does not offer any conclusions about these questions, only a plurality of particular experiences that open up new avenues of thought for spectators to explore.

The stacking of dramaturgical layer onto dramaturgical layer, of one dance followed by the next, of each song followed by another, leads to a complex web of meanings with which the spectator is invited to engage.

More than once, certain dramaturgical elements signal that perhaps the work may be coming to an end. Towards the end of the work, the spectator's mind is getting tired from the barrage of images, texts, songs, movements and languages. My mind is ready to take a rest, absorb and digest all these layers of meaning, to let everything sink in and slot into place. Still, new elements are introduced. Willkie sings Sam Brown's 'Stop', accompanied by the cello in the blues style. Wilderijkx lip-syncs along in front of the microphone, performing gestures that visualise the lyrics. Neyskens leans against the platform on which Dieltiens is sitting and also lip-syncs and visualises the lyrics of Willkie's song with gestures. Each performer seems lost in their own little world, with very little connection to each other, tired and drained.

After the final story, told by Konjar in Slovenian, the cello recommences. A goat bleats and, a few moments later, enters through the door. The opening scene talked of the killing of a goat, and this notion was revisited in the middle of the work in another story about a goat being on the back of a van. Hearing and seeing a live goat at the end of the work enables spectators to remember and connect these elements in the dramaturgical engagement with the work's content. The lights fade out to almost complete darkness, while Dieltiens has the final 'word' with his cello music.

In a series of articles published in *Tulane Drama Review*, the Italian theatre director and writer Eugenio Barba, who in the latter half of the twentieth century worked in Denmark, Norway, Poland and India, introduces the metaphor of dramaturgy as a 'weaving together' of elements, including the vocal and physical score performed by the actor, music, costumes and props (Turner & Behrndt 31). For Barba, dramaturgy can be understood as 'the overall texture that is created by the relationships and interaction between elements in a performance (Turner & Behrndt 31). Cindy Brizell and André Lepecki, editors of special issue on dramaturgy of *Women & Performance: A Journal of Feminist Theory*, also refer to dramaturgy as a 'labor of weaving together [...] text and texture, world and stage, presence and representation' (Brizzell & Lepecki 15–16).

Within this understanding of dramaturgy, Barba further emphasises the possibility of a 'simultaneous plot structure', which 'ignores linearity in favour of having several actions taking place at the same time, without regard for their causal relationship' (Watson qtd. in Turner & Behrndt 31). Again, this simultaneous mise-en-scène is characteristic of Cherkaoui's work. In *Rien de Rien*, as in subsequent works, Cherkaoui actively stages complexity in his dramaturgies, in which he accumulates disparate layers of meaning with which spectators are invited to engage. These meanings evoked by the theatrical imagery then are transcultural and intent on destabilising fixed notions about culture, nation, religion and language and Eurocentric perspectives.

Towards a Dramaturgically Engaged Spectatorship

At the end of the first decade of the twenty-first century, a special issue of *Performance Research* 'On Dramaturgy', edited by Karoline Gritzner, Patrick Primavesi and Heike Roms, set out to examine and redefine the role of the dramaturg in a changing theatre landscape that is increasingly characterised by collective creation including dance, performance art and media. The editors also drew attention to the emergence of 'new dramaturgies of the spectator', for example the article by Katia Arfara on the work of Rimini Protokoll. This, however, is a kind of theatre that relies heavily on active participation of the spectator, and therefore, it is almost implied that these dramaturgies of the spectator are reserved for participatory and interactive theatre. As will be discussed later, Van Kerkhoven's notion of a dramaturgy of the spectator refers to all theatre, including the kind of theatre that does not challenge the conventional spatial relationship between performers and audience in the proscenium arch theatre, which includes much of Cherkaoui's dance theatre.

This book articulates the role of the spectator in dance dramaturgy, as a continuous engagement with the work's lingering content, imagery, aural landscape, stories and poignant moments, which extends far beyond the performance moment. Emphasising the continuous dramaturgical work of the spectator, this book addresses a gap in the existing discourses on dance dramaturgy, which tend to focus on creative process and the role of the dramaturg in collaborative arrangements. Calls have been made to expand the notion of dramaturgy to embrace the spectator's analytical engagement with the work in order for theatre and performance to fulfil their potential for social change (Van Kerkhoven); however, not many publications frame the spectator's labour as dramaturgical. This book takes on the challenge of refining and re-defining the role of the spectator as a dramaturgical agent, particularly in relation to Cherkaoui's work.

Generally, dramaturgical practice is still largely considered as taking place before the premiere of a work, or before the performance. In this section, I will argue that the practice of dramaturgy continues beyond this point on the part of the spectator. A continuous dramaturgy of the spectator would begin to account for the continued engagement by the spectator with the work, beyond the moment of the performance itself.

> Barba sees the performance as 'the beginning of a longer experience' (Barba, 1990: 98) for the spectator. As spectators, we may not have been able to follow all the possible readings available in a performance in the moment of its performance, but we may reflect on it for months, even years, after the performance. (Turner 32)

Examples of this kind of dramaturgically engaged spectatorship are at the heart of this research. My analysis of Cherkaoui's works results from multiple viewings of the live works, close examination of a number of video recordings of the works and research of the music and the lyrics with any commercially available CDs. Over several years, a renewed engagement with the works has meant my understanding of the works' dramaturgies changed and deepened with each viewing and with each conversation about the work. I noticed elements which I had not noticed before in the dense mise-en-scène, characterised by simultaneity. Although multiple viewings of the works are not a condition for the continuous dramaturgy of the spectator, they tend to characterise the engagement of the scholar with the work. This scholarly work can be considered as a single iteration of how the continuous dramaturgy of the spectator might manifest itself.

Crucially, Van Kerkhoven establishes the need for a more profound relationship between theatre and its audiences, in order for theatre to effectuate its potential for social change, which she terms a 'macro dramaturgy of the social' (Van Kerkhoven 'Grote Dramaturgie' 69). Van Kerkhoven distinguishes between 'micro dramaturgy', localised within and around one specific production—and the main focus of the discourses on new dramaturgies—and 'macro dramaturgy'[8] or the dramaturgical activity through which theatre executes its function in society. She argues that the instantaneity of performance and its direct interaction with an audience allows theatre to develop a link with and reflect critically on society. With the aid of dramaturgy 'artists can help us to read the world, to decipher its complexity'[9] (Van Kerkhoven 'Grote Dramaturgie' 69).

However, the social potential of theatre as a straightforward process is contested and dismissed as utopian. Indeed, Van Kerkhoven does not explain what the 'macro dramaturgy of the social' entails or how it works exactly, and her argument may not fully persuade those who critically evaluate the possibility of theatre to effectuate change in society. In his article 'Towards an Expanded Dramaturgical Practice', Peter Eckersall can be seen to marry the concepts of 'micro' and 'macro dramaturgy', indicating that the two are inherently connected. He reports on his and his colleagues' initiative, the Dramaturgies forum, which investigated issues in Australian professional dramaturgical practice. This double dramaturgical practice can be seen to hold similarities with Cherkaoui's, as his new dramaturgy is also rooted in the postdramatic theatrical field and the context of neoliberal capitalism. The key argument of Eckersall's text is that dramaturgy itself is a process that thrives on a state of 'creative indecision', a strategic 'refusal and resistance to closure', which is deemed reflective of this wider context (Eckersall 284–285). 'The uncomfortable relationship that dramaturgy has in the theatrical process, and the discomfort sometimes experienced by dramaturgs as their role is questioned, might be seen as productive, if not a measure of the dramaturgical process as a whole' (Eckersall 295). The concept of an 'expanded dramaturgical practice' is based on the notion of dramaturgy as 'a tool to challenge cultural norms and established systems of production while also aiding in their realization and further development' (Eckersall 285). While this is a useful way of conceiving of macro dramaturgy beyond the immediate micro-dramaturgical, theatrical context by moving into the wider cultural arena, there are some limitations to Eckersall's project. In the context of Eckersall's research, dramaturgy is mainly conceived of as the work of the dramaturg as an individual, collaborating with the artist, and not the wider practice that includes non-professionals I am suggesting here. While Eckersall does emphasise that, in order for theatre to 'work effectively', it is necessary to 'conspicuously invit[e] a sense of dialogue and engagement with the audience that requires their overt participation in the making of theatre' (Eckersall 294), this comment comes right at the end of his article. Eckersall's notion does not fully explore the involvement of the spectator in effecting the challenging of cultural norms through engaging with the theatrical work in an extended macro-dramaturgical practice, which I argue is a crucial step in completing the dramaturgical project. Therefore, the expanded macro dramaturgy suggested by Eckersall, and its potential to effect change and cultural intervention, would need to be extended further by articulating and emphasising the role of the spectator.

Barba's notion of the dramaturgy of the spectator began to articulate dramaturgy as a labour that is not confined to the professional labour of the dramaturg. However, like the dramaturgy of the actor, it needs extension. The actor's dramaturgy stipulates that each participant in the creative process takes responsibility through improvisation and a refining of the actor's score, a process considered congruous with the notion of shared dramaturgical responsibility and a micro-dramaturgical context. Likewise, the spectator is considered to be an important agent in the dramaturgical process too, as illustrated in this lengthy quote from Turner's summary:

> The spectator's dramaturgy is constructed through the experience of the performance, the connection that each individual makes in relation to the many threads that are woven together by the performers to create a sense of coherence. A performance should not intend to make a meaning explicit but should intend to create spaces where the spectator may question the potential and available meanings in the performance. (Turner 32)

Returning to another of Van Kerkhoven's texts, in her contribution to the special issue of *Performance Research* 'On Dramaturgy', she explained that in order to engage with the notion of European dramaturgy there is need for a

> focus on [...] the actual relationship of the artist with this world, on the dialogue, that is or could be held between the artwork and the audience, on the relationship between theatre-practice and its theoretical questioners, on the conversations we have to carry on with or about Europe etc. (Van Kerkhoven 'European Dramaturgy' 7)

She made reference to the 'emancipation of the spectator' without explicitly citing Rancière's text, in order to account for the labour of the spectator in constructing meaning from the various fragments that make up a performance. She considered the increasing mediatisation of culture to be problematic as it limits the possibility of critical perspectives, a 'de-politicization of our looking' (Van Kerkhoven 'European Dramaturgy' 11). 'In theatre, however, there remains an opening, a chance to reconquer the political countervoice, the voice of the reflecting individual' (Van Kerkhoven 'European Dramaturgy' 11). Van Kerkhoven's was one of the only voices in the Anglophone discourse on new dramaturgies that explicitly drew attention to the role of the spectator in dramaturgy and hence moved the discourse beyond the need to articulate the role of the professional dramaturg. She emphasised the importance of conversation when specifying what this macro-dramaturgical labour of the spectator might entail:

> Dramaturgy is for me learning to handle complexity. It is feeding the ongoing conversation on the work, it is taking care of the reflexive potential [...] Dramaturgy is building bridges, it is being responsible for the whole, dramaturgy is above all a constant movement. Inside and outside. The readiness to dive into the work, and to withdraw from it again and again, inside, outside, trampling the leaves. A constant movement. (Van Kerkhoven 'European Dramaturgy' 11)

Van Kerkhoven indicated a tenacious engagement with the work on behalf of the spectator, an ongoing and continuous labour that extends far beyond the moment of the performance. This kind of labour might traditionally be found in academic scholarship on dance and theatre, but has not explicitly been acknowledged as being in effect dramaturgical. This is, in essence, one of the main arguments of this book: that the scholarly labour on dance and theatre is recognised as dramaturgical. In order for dramaturgy to fulfil its potential to impact on the social, and challenge cultural norms, it must extend to include the spectator and continue beyond the performance event itself.

NOTES

1. Laermans and Gielen frame 'the Flemish dance wave' as a concept through which the artists involved constructed identities. They argue that the coincidence of the disparate figures in the Flemish contemporary dance field— Anne Teresa De Keersmaeker, Jan Fabre and Wim Vandekeybus—was deliberately constructed as 'the Flemish dance wave', notwithstanding and perhaps despite the lack of stable funding structures for the art form. The term 'wave' meant that the artists involved could cause a greater impact

abroad and mobilise this influence at home to legitimise their work and over time unlock more stable funding arrangements.

2. The translation of Van Kerkhoven's original Dutch text into the three other languages shows a few flaws and inconsistencies. In the Dutch original and German translations, both of the gendered pronouns (respectively *hij/zij* and *er/sie*) are used consistently to indicate the dramaturg. However, in the English and French translations, sometimes only the masculine pronouns (respectively *he* and *il*) are used. This apparent neglect and lack of awareness of feminist issues surrounding the writing raises questions about the reliability of the translations. The translation of the Dutch phrase 'het geheel' into the English word 'global' also raises doubt. The Dutch word 'globaal' is often used in relation to the notion of entirety, to which this paragraph refers. The English word 'global', however, is mostly used to refer to the world.

3. Guy Cools too, in his role of Cherkaoui's dramaturg, has become increasingly visible over the years. His voice as the dramaturg is expressed in programme leaflets, pre- or post-performance talks with audiences and discussions.

4. 'interlocuteur'.

5. 'legitimering en didactiek'.

6. 'de dramaturg belichaamt het gebrek'.

7. The only exception in the 2000–2010 period may be *Sutra*, where the more homogenous score is composed by Szymon Brzóska and there is no spoken word.

8. 'kleine' and 'grote dramaturgie', in line with Lepecki's in deLahunta.

9. 'kunstenaars kunnen ons helpen de wereld te lezen, zijn complexiteit te ontcijferen'.

BIBLIOGRAPHY

Arfara, Katia. 'Aspects of a New Dramaturgy of the Spectator'. *Performance Research*. 14.3. (2009): 112–118. Print.

Barba, Eugenio. *On Directing and Dramaturgy: Burning the House*. Oxon: Routledge, 2009. Print.

Brizzell, Cindy & Lepecki, André. 'Introduction: The Labor of the Question Is the (Feminist) Question of Dramaturgy'. *Women & Performance: A Journal of Feminist Theory*. 26.13:2. (2003): 15–16. Print.

Contemporary Theatre Review. Issue on 'New Dramaturgies'. Turner, Cathy & Behrndt, Synne. Eds. 20:2. (2010). Print.

Cvejić, Bojana. 'The Ignorant Dramaturg'. *Maska*. 16.131–132. (2010): 40–53. Print.

deLahunta, Scott. 'Dance Dramaturgy: Speculations and Reflections'. *Dance Theatre Journal*. 16.1. (2000): 20–25. Print.

deLahunta, Scott; Ginot, Isabelle; Lepecki, André; Rethorst, Susan; Theodores, Diana; Van Imschoot, Myriam & Williams, David. 'Conversations on Choreography'. *Performance Research*. 8.4. (2003): 61–70.

De Laet, Timmy. 'Giving Sense to the Past: Historical D(is)ance and the Chiasmatic Interlacing of Affect and Knowledge'. *The Oxford Handbook of Dance and Reenactment*. Ed. Franko, Mark. Oxford: Oxford University Press, 2017. 33–56. Print.

De Vuyst, Hildegard. 'Een Dramaturgie Van Het Gebrek: Paradoxen en Dubbelzinnigheden'.*Etcetera*. 17.68. (1999): 65–66. Print.

Eckersall, Peter. 'Towards an Expanded Dramaturgical Practice: A Report on "The Dramaturgy and Cultural Intervention Project"'. *Theatre Research International*. 31.3. (2006): 283–297. Print.

Gregg, Melissa & Seigworth, Gregory J. Eds. *The Affect Theory Reader*. Durham, NC: Duke University Press, 2010. Print.

Hansen, Pil & Callison, Darcey. *Dance Dramaturgy: Modes of Agency, Awareness and Engagement*. New World Choreographies Series. London: Palgrave Macmillan, 2015. Print.

Kealiinohomoku, Joann. 'An Anthropologist Looks at Ballet as a Form of Ethnic Dance'. *What Is Dance? Readings in Theory and Criticism*. Ed. Copeland, Roger & Cohen, Marshall. Oxford: Oxford University Press, 1983. 533–549. Print.

Khoury, Krystel. 'Un arbre aux possibilités multiples: Le traitement de la main dans le travail chorégraphique de Sidi Larbi Cherkaoui'. *Des mains modernes: Cinéma, danse, photographie, théâtre*. Ed. André, Emmanuelle; Claudia Palazzolo & Emmanuel Siety. Paris: L'Harmattan, 2008. 14–26. Print.

Laermans, Rudi & Gielen, Pascal. 'Flanders—Constructing Identities: The Case of "the Flemish Dance Wave"'. *Europe Dancing: Perspectives on Theatre Dance and Cultural Identity*. Ed. Grau, Andrée & Jordan, Stephanie. London: Routledge, 2000. 12–27. Print.

Ong, Walter. *Orality and Literacy: The Technologizing of the Word*. 2nd Ed. New York: Routledge, 2002. Print.

Performance Research. Issue 'On Dramaturgy'. Gritzner, Karoline; Primavesi, Patrick & Roms, Heike. Eds. 14:3. (2009). Print.

Rancière, Jacques. *The Emancipated Spectator*. London: Verso, 2009. Print.

Turner, Cathy & Behrndt, Synne. *Dramaturgy and Performance*. Basingstoke: Palgrave Macmillan, 2008. Print.

Turner, Jane. *Eugenio Barba*. Routledge Performance Practitioners Series. Oxon: Routledge, 2004. Print.

Van Heuven, Robbert. 'De Dramaturg #2: Marianne Van Kerkhoven: "Dramaturgie is de bezielde structuur van de voorstelling"'. *TM: Tijdschrift over Theater, Muziek en Dans.* 9.8. (2005): 16–18. Print.

Van Imschoot, Myriam. 'Anxious Dramaturgy'. *Women & Performance: A Journal of Feminist Theory.* 26.13:2. (2003): 57–68. Print.

Van Kerkhoven, Marianne. 'Looking Without Pencil in the Hand'. *Theaterschrift.* 5–6. (1994). 140–148. Print.

———. 'Van de Kleine en Grote Dramaturgie: Pleidooi voor een "Interlocuteur"'. *Etcetera.* 17.68. (1999): 67–69. Print.

———. 'European Dramaturgy in the 21st Century'. *Performance Research.* 14.3. (2009): 7–11. Print.

Wehrs, Donald R. & Blake, Thomas. Eds. *The Palgrave Handbook of Affect Studies and Textual Criticism.* London: Palgrave Macmillan, 2017. Print.

Multimedia Source

Rien de Rien. Choreographed by Sidi Larbi Cherkaoui. 2000. Video Recording of Performance.

CHAPTER 3

Transculturality and Its Limits in *Zero Degrees* and *Sutra*

Beyond academic discourses foregrounding cultural hybridity, general notions of culture as 'discrete entities with impermeable boundaries, ... defined by the borders of the nation-state' still loom large in the twenty-first century (Bond & Rapson 7). Indeed, political movements such as the Flemish populist radical right around the turn of the millennium, discussed in the introduction as the contextual backdrop to the emergence of Cherkaoui's choreographic work, continue to illustrate these hegemonic ways of thinking that originated during the Enlightenment. In *zero degrees* (2005), Cherkaoui and his co-choreographer and co-performer Akram Khan, directly tackle these colonial conceptions of the nation as a container of culture, instead exploring transculturality and exposing the nation for its constructed nature. It is a work that has received both public acclaim and scholarly attention (Khoury; Mitra; Cools; Sörgel). At the end of this chapter, I offer a brief study of Cherkaoui's work *Sutra* (2008), made in collaboration with monks of the Shaolin Temple. The work is read as an ethnographic exploration that tests the limits of Cherkaoui's transcultural choreographic project.

The title *zero degrees* refers to the "in between" point, the point between positive and negative, between water and ice, between life and death, between one state boundary and the other, between performance and visual arts. The dramaturgical focus is on the moment when one thing becomes another, the moment of transformation. Dance and theatre scholar Royona Mitra, in her astute reading of *zero degrees* through

© The Author(s) 2019
L. Uytterhoeven, *Sidi Larbi Cherkaoui*, New World Choreographies,
https://doi.org/10.1007/978-3-030-27816-8_3

the influential postcolonial lens of Homi K. Bhabha's notions of hybridity and third space, equally identifies that the work brings to the fore new ways of choreographing diaspora and cultural identity. She coins the notion of 'new interculturalism' in relation to Khan's work more broadly, highlighting Khan's 'perpetual identification with a state of in-betweenness; between cultures, between nations, between disciplines and between the different versions of his own self, with a recognition that many selves and many others coexist within him' (Mitra 29). It is argued that Khan's interrogation of the process of othering from the very perspective of the Other blurs 'simplistic categories' like 'us' and 'them' (Mitra 30). However, when reflecting on Cherkaoui's dramaturgical contribution to *zero degrees*, transculturalism seems more apt as a lens through which to examine the work in relation to his larger choreographic oeuvre in comparison with interculturalism. Whereas Khan's starting point is that of 'auto-ethnography', a 'self-referential enquiry [...] through which he tries to raise questions about himself' (Mitra 29), Cherkaoui's starting point is one of transformation, becoming the Other. It seems that Khan's position is introspective, whereas Cherkaoui's driving force is one of reaching out, collaborating and connecting with others. The resulting transformation of both the self, the collaborators and, eventually, also the spectator, parallels the concept of transculturality.

With regard to hybridity, the focus in Bhabha's essay 'Culture In-Between', like it is in *zero degrees*, is on 'the contaminated yet connective tissue between cultures – at once the possibility of culture's connectedness and the border between them'. Bhabha envisions the collision of 'part' or 'partial' cultures in the colonial context as 'pregnant with the potential for new world visions'. Artists such as Cherkaoui and Khan can be classed as using their postcolonial subjectivity through a kind of 'interstitial agency that refuses the binary representation of social antagonism'. These kinds of 'hybrid agencies [...] deploy the partial culture from which they emerge to construct visions of community, and versions of historic memory, that give narrative form to the minority positions they occupy'. However, in this chapter, it will be explored to what extent Cherkaoui may be considered to exceed this kind of hybrid agency and transforms it into a transcultural and cosmopolitan agency through his larger dramaturgic project, which seeks out and choreographs partiality and sharedness in all cultural encounters.

THE TRANSCULTURAL PERSPECTIVE

In situating the term transcultural within the intellectual context in which it gained and, to an extent, lost traction, I draw on perspectives from cultural, media and literary studies, as well as scholarly work on cultural memory. When attempting to formulate a working definition of the term transcultural, most simply put it refers to 'a more fluid and transient paradigm of relations between societies', which entails a rejection of a 'bordered' and 'fixed' understanding of culture (Bond & Rapson 9). Transculturality oscillates between the local and the global. The scholar who instigated an interest in transculturality is Wolfgang Welsch, working in the field of aesthetics. His point of departure is a resolute critique of the traditional concept of single cultures, which he concludes is predicated on the simultaneous processes of 'inner homogenization' and 'exclusion of the foreign'. Moreover, conceiving of cultures as singular does not account for their inner complexity, cutting across differences in social class, gender and sexuality. He posits that 'the purity precept renders impossible a mutual understanding between cultures' and that, although rooted in the fiction that cultures would not intermingle, in practice, the notion becomes 'politically dangerous' and 'untenable'. The alternative conceptions of multiculturalism and interculturalism go some way towards accounting for plurality but are rejected by Welsch because they still presuppose the traditional concept of single cultures as islands or spheres. Transculturality, in contrast, enables cultural observers to account for cultures' entanglement, mixedness and permeability.

> It is a matter of readjusting our inner compass: away from the concentration on the polarity of the own and the foreign to an attentiveness for what might be common and connective wherever we encounter things foreign. (Welsch)

Welsch contends that transculturality does not result in increasing homogeneisation, but in diversity and plurality, referring to these networks as 'transcultural webs [...] which have some things in common while differing in others, showing overlaps and distinctions at the same time'. These transcultural networks can instead be visualised well through the image of the kaleidoscope, already invoked by Justin Morin in relation to Cherkaoui as 'l'homme kaleidoscope'. For Welsch, the static image of the mosaic, often invoked in multiculturalism, is no longer an adequate visualisation since it presupposes 'a juxtaposition of clearly delineated cultures'. Instead, the moving images of the kaleidoscope lend themselves well to the transcultural conception that cultures and identities are constantly shifting and changing, blending into one another, always in process and never fixed.

Critiques of transculturality include the thought that this way of thinking is too much of an abstraction, which denies historical specificity and leads to vagueness, rather than shedding light on particular relationships of cultural indebtedness (Tutek). 'One should be blunt and say that the friction [between cultural groups] comes about as a function of the global production of inequality that puts certain populations and their cultures in a position of perpetual material dependency that gives birth to an understandable bitterness, anxiety, and resistance (both on their part and on the part of the ones in more privileged positions) which cannot simply be removed culturally — by fostering understanding or offering more open models of cultural analysis — because the cultures themselves are forged from this inequality' (Tutek). Perhaps one of the reasons why transculturality has not caught on as a concept in fields that are not applied, like it is, for example, in transcultural education or social care, is that it is deemed too idealistic and utopian. These critiques rightly stipulate that transculturality is not going to redress global inequalities shaped by centuries of colonialism and capitalism. However, I would still like to advocate for a continued engagement with transculturality, as it would not do harm to entertain its possibility as a useful concept. Moreover, perhaps the concept is visionary, but its promise as yet unfulfilled. As the notion of 'trans-' has gained more traction in recent years, we might also begin to see changes in popular conceptions of culture, away from nationalism and towards transcultural ways of thinking.

Dance and theatre scholar Rachel Fensham and Odette Kelada, a scholar in creative writing, culture and communication, emphasise the potential of transculturality for, through and beyond dance, precisely because of its foregrounding of movement. 'The term describes interconnection and entanglement ensuing from various forces including migratory processes to communication systems and economic interdependencies' (Fensham & Kelada 366). It enables a taking account of the inner complexity of the dancing body, its corporeality. As such, dance as a scholarly discipline can act as a catalyst for broader investigations into transcultural experience, forging new understandings of identity, away from monolithic categories such as the nation.

COLLABORATIVE CREATIVE PROCESSES IN *ZERO DEGREES*

In this section, I will analyse *zero degrees* by introducing the contributions to the creative process made by each of Cherkaoui's collaborators. First and foremost, Cherkaoui's co-choreographer and co-performer in this work is Akram Khan. In fact, their meeting in Belgium at P.A.R.T.S., resulting friendship and subsequent desire to work together was the raison d'être for *zero degrees*. The movement material in the work is a direct result of this exchange, strongly influenced by Khan's virtuosity in Kathak, which he shared with Cherkaoui through daily morning practice. However, the joint aim of the endeavour is not to 'invent a new choreographic language' or to 'blend and fuse their artistic identities'; instead, through an episodic structure in which solos, duets and storytelling scenes follow each other, Cherkaoui and Khan 'choose – already in *zero degrees* – to juxtapose them, letting them coexist' (Cools 79–80).

The dramaturgical backbone of the work is a travel story, which Khan told Cherkaoui early on in the process and which is meticulously rehearsed, reproduced and performed in unison by the two performers. The significance of this and other travel stories in Cherkaoui's work will be analysed in the next sections. However, to give a further impression of the movement material in *zero degrees*, it is possible to discern a visualising of certain kinetic elements in the story through choreographed material. For example, in the story, a train journey is mentioned, and the danced scene that follows visualises the motion of a train on the tracks, aided by percussive, repetitive music, based on syncopated rhythms. The pair's stomping feet trace a triangular pattern, wide in front of the body, narrow at the back. Their arms swing powerfully forwards and backwards, hands slightly crossing in front of the body, slicing through the air surrounding the body. While the arms swing back, the legs move forward, in perfect opposition. This pattern is repeated endlessly, mechanically and as if powered by an outside force. While, in its most basic form, the pair perform it stationary facing towards the audience, they also use it to travel, mostly maintaining the forward-facing orientation of the body. Almost as soon as a pattern of unison is established, it is abandoned as Cherkaoui and Khan begin to slightly and loosely shift the rhythm, so they fall in and out of sync, as if they are testing where the potential alignment of their identities begins and ends. Later, they play with the movement even more freely, simply keeping the downbeat stomping as an anchor, while they spin, fall, roll, arch back, jump, drop to their knees and twist.

Both in the movement material generated in the context of the work and that more closely derived from traditional Kathak, Cherkaoui's embodiment is very different from Khan's. Indeed, their bodies are very different: Cherkaoui being tall, pale and very lean and Khan being compact, brown-skinned and sturdy. However, it would not be just to essentialise these bodies and the way they move, ignoring the impact of daily training practices on the dancers' physicality. Cherkaoui struggles with the down-jumps and groundedness required, while Khan's dancing body does not lend itself well to high extensions of the limbs that characterise Cherkaoui's style. However, the latter are much avoided in the shared choreography; hence, it seems that Cherkaoui is making himself more vulnerable in performance by revealing the limitations of his skill as a dancer compared to Khan. It may even be said that this exploration of the limits of his skills is a driving force for Cherkaoui. Since *zero degrees*, he pursued two further duets in which he transforms into the Other, setting out to 'consciously […] study another dance language' (Cools). In *Dunas* (2009), co-created with celebrated flamenco dancer María Pagés, he tries on her movement. Critics, however, were not altogether impressed. The two dancers are described as 'dynamic opposites' and stating that Cherkaoui 'lacks the authentic flamenco hauteur' (Gilbert). Another review is focused on the idea that 'their exchange has a one-way character' and that the work is merely 'an exhibition […] of his imitative skills' (Jennings). Perhaps it should be considered that Cherkaoui is not necessarily focused on achieving what critics describe as 'choreographic rigour' (Jennings), but on the embodied exploration of transcultural networks through collaboration as an end in and of itself. The very notion of 'rigour', a word that carries the etymological connotation of stiffness within it, seems incompatible with Cherkaoui's larger project. Another noteworthy duet pursued by Cherkaoui following *zero degrees* is *Play* (2010), with Kuchipudi dancer Shantala Shivalingappa.

Other movement influences in *zero degrees* are that of Hatha Yoga, through Cherkaoui's collaboration with Sri Louise, who acted as a physical coach during the process. In a solo, during which Cherkaoui displays extreme virtuosity of his own, his increased strength is visible in the measured execution of headstands, which from time to time morph into shoulder stands while his back is arched and his legs are bent over his torso. The hypermobility of Cherkaoui's body is harnessed in *zero degrees* to create contortionist poses; for example, one leg is folded over his head and, with his arm hooked behind his leg, he strokes his beard. Another movement influence is Kung Fu, visible in a sparring duet between Cherkaoui and Khan. They thrust extended palms into each other's negative space, in other words, the space immediately surrounding their body or the space in which their body is not. They react to each other's intended blows by dodging them and blocking them off with raised forearms, letting these martial arts movements lead them into freer dance movement sequences. Following this brief exploration of Kung Fu in *zero degrees*, Cherkaoui later pursued his interest in this martial art form and transcultural dramaturgy further through *Sutra*, discussed in the final section of this chapter.

The collaboration with Turner-prize winning visual artist Antony Gormley on the design for *zero degrees* is made visible in the two white, life-size, latex casts of the dancers' bodies, who join them on stage. Gormley, a sculptor who has pursued a lifelong interest in the body, most notably his own body, has developed a practice of making casts of his body, which he positions in different locations, both natural and urban. The documentary *zero degrees: L'Infini* by French filmmaker Gilles Delmas captured the process of making the casts of dancers' bodies, also referred to as "dummies", given that they resemble crash-test dummies. In a claustrophobic process, having only a little straw through which to breathe, the body is enveloped in a material that takes a while to set. This is a further correlation with the title of the work: the negative space around the body is positivised and used to create casts of the body. The interface where skin meets substance is hence the zero degree point. Cherkaoui admits that the confrontation with the cast of his body, a representation of his body in three dimensions, was very unsettling and very different from seeing the body reflected in two dimensions in a mirror (*zero degrees* DVD). The cast of Cherkaoui's body has an internal skeleton and is hence able to stand upright, while the shoulder joints are mobile. The cast of Khan's body, however, can articulate almost all of it joints and, in the absence of a skeleton, is hence incapable of standing up. This is perhaps an inversion of the respective strength and hypermobility of the two performers themselves. Recalling the ways in which Cherkaoui began to explore puppet-like manipulations of bodies in *Rien de Rien*, the fact that in *zero degrees* he and Khan are joined by two actual puppets, duplications of their own bodies, multiplies the possibilities of both choreographic play and a continued dramaturgical exploration of power and manipulation.

There are two defining scenes in the work that involve the puppets. The first shows Cherkaoui faced with his dummy centre stage. He manipulates the dummy's arms to suggest that they are exchanging gestures of greeting and friendship, such as shaking hands and patting each other on the shoulder. Soon, though, a slight inflection of narcissistic or homoerotic tension—the dummy "strokes" Cherkaoui's cheek—is followed by aggression. The stroking suddenly turns into a slap across the face. The dummy pounds Cherkaoui's head until he is kneeling, carefully glancing up at his aggressor, terrorised. Autobiographical elements come to my mind, in the sense that Cherkaoui's homosexuality was taboo for his father and as a result this repression may have been internalised. Cherkaoui has indicated in interview that this scene stems from the idea of seeking self-acceptance. After the power struggle with the puppet escalates to a strangling gesture, reminiscent of the type of strangling the popular cartoon character Homer Simpson is quick to resort to in dealing with his son, Cherkaoui is still reaching out to his Other. To conclude the scene and put an end to the ridiculous suspension of disbelief[1] he has seduced the spectator into, Cherkaoui climbs into the arms of the dummy, expecting it to hold and carry him in front of its chest. To a tragicomic effect, the puppet falls backwards and Cherkaoui lands on top of it.

A second key scene involving the dummies shows Khan and the latex cast of his body lying face down on the floor, with Khan assuming almost the exact same position as his puppet. The way in which he ended up there is significant: Khan moves across the stage, his steps growing increasingly larger, until he almost does the splits and falls down. He glances over at his dummy and gathers himself, only to fall back down, as if he is tripped by an invisible force. These glances continue, as if Khan knows that it is inevitable that he will end up being on the floor just like his puppet. However, he keeps pulling himself out of the floor, only to be thrust back down, until he finally gives up and his body has seemingly lost all power and agency. Cherkaoui walks over and surveys the situation, hands on hips, taking in the similarity of the positions occupied by Khan and his puppet. The only dissimilarity is the way the head is turned. So, Cherkaoui flips Khan's head with his foot, indicating that Khan's body is now an object that does not warrant even the least amount of respect. Walking over to the dummy, Cherkaoui wipes the sweat off his face in a working man's gesture, and stamps down hard on the middle of the dummy's back, resembling the action of starting an old-timer car. Khan exaggerates the reaction of the blow in his own body, as if he and the dummy are one and the same. By manipulating the dummy, Cherkaoui is able to control Khan's body too. He quickly repeats the same action again, met by the same reaction in Khan's body, and follows up with dragging the puppet across a little by the arm. Khan also moves across a little. Cherkaoui touches his chin, pensively. He kicks the side of the ribcage, the hand and the head. He grabs hold of the head with both hands and twists the neck forcibly from side to side. He drags the dummy by the hand onto its back. Khan does the same but in the opposite direction. Cherkaoui is left standing in the middle, bewildered. In a further cartoonesque game with the suspension of disbelief, Cherkaoui lifts up Khan's hand, looking at the dummy's lifeless arm left on the floor, expecting it to react like Khan had before. Giggles in the audience. Grabbing both Khan and the dummy by the hand, he drags both across the floor. I am suddenly conscious of how heavy they must be, remembering from Delmas's documentary that the puppets are not only life-size, but also made to be as heavy as the bodies from which they are cast. Cherkaoui lifts both Khan and the dummy onto his shoulder and then suddenly drops them. He connects Khan's hand with the dummy's and drags both of them by the puppet's other hand, until he is near the standing cast of his own body. He reaches out to it, expecting it to grab onto his hand, but again, the same joke has not yet got old. Finally reaching over and grabbing his dummy's hand, to which it falls forward onto the ground, Cherkaoui is the only one left standing in a chain of four, edging forward but stuck because the lifeless bodies are weighing him down. He drags his dummy over to the other side of the chain and connects Khan's free hand with the other dummy. Now Cherkaoui can use both hands and his own body weight to drag the chain across the floor. He reaches out to the side, but there is no one there to pull him; then, he looks into the audience and reaches out to them. Nobody is laughing. He props his dummy onto its feet and reconnects Khan's hand to it. He wanders over to the other side of the chain, looks around, scratches his head and then drops to the floor, his hand grabbing Khan's dummy's on the floor. The image is a reversal of the previous chain, the dummy now standing up and Cherkaoui now lying down. Spectators laugh again (Fig. 3.1).

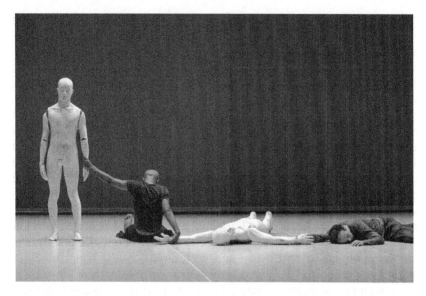

Fig. 3.1   Akram Khan and Sidi Larbi Cherkaoui in *zero degrees* (Photo by Agathe Poupeney)

In this scene, Khan puts himself "in the shoes" of his dummy and visualises the impact of the blows his duplicate receives. This exaggerated and absurd display of embodied empathy puzzles and confuses Cherkaoui, who experiments further, testing which body is able to perform which actions. In these interactions, the initial violence indirectly inflected upon Khan's body through Cherkaoui's kicking of the dummy gives way to absurd tragicomedy. Cherkaoui proves himself to be a poor and ineffective manipulator of other bodies. He is ultimately unable to coerce the bodies into submission, and he is literally dragged down by their weight. A game is being played here with the ideas of transformation into the Other and the limits of empathy. Cherkaoui's reaching out to the audience at the end of the scene may seem fruitless at first glance. However, this gesture directly aimed at the people in the auditorium jolts them into reflection, about who needs help and why, who is in a position to help and how, and whether they should help or do nothing. This is a choreographic and dramaturgic reiteration of a moment in the travel story recounted by Khan and Cherkaoui throughout the work, about a woman on a train needing help with the body of her dead husband. The dramaturgic implications of this travel story will be discussed in more detail later in this chapter; however, Cherkaoui's gesture reaching out for help serves to cement this notion as a dramaturgic red thread in the work.

Mikki Kunttu's lighting design adds to the multiplication of bodily figures on stage through the creation of shadows. In a scene towards the beginning of the work, the two dancers travel from side to side whilst first spinning one way, then the other. A set of two shadows is created on each of the three tall, white walls surrounding them, which make the stage space resemble that of a white-space gallery. The stark design aesthetics of this work are a marked contrast to the warm and busy atmosphere of Cherkaoui's previous works, in which the stage was often layered with raised platforms and filled with objects and props. Notably, the musicians, performing live, as is one of Cherkaoui's core artistic values, are not visually integrated on stage as they were in *Rien de Rien*, *Foi* and *Tempus Fugit*; instead, they are separated from the onstage action by the large, white, semi-translucent cyc at the back of the stage space. When I first saw *zero degrees* in 2005, this visual design was one of the largest contrasts between this and Cherkaoui's previous works, directly resulting from the collaboration with Khan, Gormley and Kunttu and hence marking a new line of artistic and aesthetic inquiry for Cherkaoui.

As Cherkaoui and Khan move, some shadows become larger while others diminish over time, and then back again. At times, the shadows overlap, suggesting a merging of the two choreographers' identities. Although at one point Cherkaoui is standing downstage right and Khan upstage left, their shadows on the back wall come together in a scene that shows Khan holding out his hand in a begging gesture and Cherkaoui reaching out to the grab the hand, only for the two performers to lean so far that they tumble sideways, destroying this momentary image.

To conclude the image of the visual design, the costumes by Japanese-born textile artist Kei Ito are also worth noting. In an interview about her practice, she indicates being interested in the juxtaposition between East and West in the way that body and fabric relate to one another (Woolf). This is visible in *zero degrees* in the design of wide-legged trousers and tight-fitting T-shirts. The trousers consist of several panels that overlap, evoking the folding of origami. As the dancers spin, the wide trousers move through space in a reactionary way. Cherkaoui wears blue and grey, while Khan wears khaki green, the only hints of colour in an otherwise white and grey space with lighting devoid of colour.

For the musical landscape in *zero degrees*, Cherkaoui and Khan collaborated with British Asian composer and musician Nitin Sawhney. A score for cello, violin, percussion and Sufi singing vocals, the music is multi-layered and complex, both rhythmically and melodically, and underscores the dramaturgical development of the work in refined ways. Perhaps representing a new juncture in the composition process for Sawhney, at the end of the work the musical score has to work around the live singing by Cherkaoui of the song 'Yerushalayim Shel Zahav', to which it adds complementing harmonies on the strings and vocals.

The final collaborative partner in *zero degrees* is Guy Cools, the dramaturg. He somewhat downplays his role on the collaboration by insisting on his role being one of merely moderating (Cools). 'The main part of my work is to listen to both [choreographers] individually expressing their concerns about the process and each other's expectations and anxieties toward it, and to moderate the discussions between them and also with the other artistic collaborators. A good moderator keeps his own voice and opinion out of the discussion' (Cools 122). In relation to transculturality, Cools posits that the value of dramaturgy lies precisely in its dialogic nature. 'A dialogical practice and attitude is fundamental to any creative process in which you want to meet and exchange with the other. It doesn't exclude misunderstandings or disagreements, but it is the only way to interweave different voices polyphonically' (Cools 123). This dramaturgical work, however invisible it may be, is absolutely crucial for the creative process. I would argue that it becomes visible in the balance of simultaneous clarity and obscurity of the dramaturgical elements in the work. Clarity comes through in the unity between the work's title, visual design and narrative elements. Obscurity exists in a number of untranslated cultural elements leading to rich macro-dramaturgical layers, some of which are only accessible to the spectator through ongoing work, conversations and personal research. As such, the dramaturgical extends beyond the creative process in which the work is generated and extends to the relationship between the work and the spectator—its analytical function—in line with Van Kerkhoven's seminal definition of the term in her 1994 essay 'Looking Without Pencil in the Hand', discussed in Chapter 2.

THE TRAVEL STORY

At the heart of *zero degrees* is a travel story told by Khan, about a journey he made to India and Bangladesh. Added to Angélique Willkie's
story in *Rien de Rien*, the inclusion of Khan's story in *zero degrees* indicates that travel stories are a key dramaturgic interest of Cherkaoui's and
were often generative creative sources for his early work. In theorising
the travel story, I will draw on both postcolonial perspectives of the
emergence of the genre in the eighteenth century (Pratt) and on Walter
Benjamin's discussion of the figure of the storyteller as a pre-modern
cultural agent.

In her book *Imperial Eyes: Travel Writing and Transculturation*, the
language and literature scholar Mary Louise Pratt provides one of the
key historical and postcolonial perspectives on the genre of the travel
story. She identifies travel writing as a key labour that aimed to natural-
ise Eurocentric world views from the eighteenth century and justify the
colonial project.

> [...] travel books written by Europeans about non-European parts of the
> world created the imperial order for Europeans "at home" and gave them
> their place in it. [...] [They] gave reading publics a sense of ownership,
> entitlement and familiarity with respect to the distant parts of the world
> [...] (Pratt 3)

She considers a wealth of writing that emerged from the mid-eighteenth
century, when attention turned from maritime to interior exploration
and a growing interest in natural history emerged. While Pratt insists
on the heterogeneity of the genre, a combining factor is that the various forms of travel stories were generated from 'contact zones' or 'social
spaces where disparate cultures meet, clash, and grapple with each other,
often in highly asymmetrical relations of domination and subordination'
(Pratt 7).

It could be argued that the concept of the contact zone can be
extended to make sense of tourism and migration in the globalised
world. In the case of Willkie's travel story in *Rien de Rien*, while issues
of power and privilege remain, the social and cultural distinctions
between coloniser and colonised are no longer clear-cut as was the case
in the eighteenth century. Willkie calls into question both the practices
of the society she visited and those of the society she belongs to and

refuses to be fully identified with either. Likewise, Khan's story reveals ambivalence in the way he identifies with both Britain and Bangladesh simultaneously, an emphasis dependent on the particular situation in which he finds himself. Due to this lack of a clear-cut and singular identity, there are limitations to the application of Pratt's historical discussion of the colonial travel story to contemporary, postcolonial travel stories. However, the concept of the contact zone remains useful to this analysis of storytelling in Cherkaoui's works, as it is argued that the contact zone is one that he actively explores and exploits when creating work.

It is worth noting that Cherkaoui seems to be mainly interested in working with individual performers who are aware of the contact zones within the Self, in other words, those performers who have a destabilised sense of Self due to a mixed cultural background or due to migration. Cherkaoui chooses deliberately to incorporate travel stories into his choreographies, as these tend to reveal cultural difference and friction as experienced by the traveller, or the contact zone within the Self. Moments when the performers grapple with these internal contact zones are highlighted in the hesitations and searching for words in their storytelling. Cherkaoui is keen to meticulously preserve and amplify these moments of hesitation by rehearsing them and continually reproducing them through performance, as opposed to smoothing them out and tidying up the text.

On his interest in storytelling and gesture as a choreographic starting point, Cherkaoui explained in an interview on the commercially available DVD of *zero degrees* that he wanted to draw attention to the small movements that accompany informal speech. 'All these things [gestures] mean something. They mean something beyond the words. So, when I started to work around the concept of theatre, next to the idea of dance, for me theatre had lacked a lot of things. It lacks the honesty of a real encounter. A real encounter, in which people don't speak with cleaned text. [A theatre text is] so cleaned up that it's not human anymore and I have a hard time listening to theatre text sometimes, because it's too clean, so it doesn't help me perceive the truth. And, so, what I like to do is film people and look at them for what they really are, how they really speak, with all the... with all the... with all the hesitations in it. With all the moments of... uh, no, and going back into the sentence, and the melody and the intonation and the way all of this is placed in itself. The way the movements are placing themselves. I think our way of talking to each other is much more than just clean words on a piece of paper' (Cherkaoui). Here, Cherkaoui firmly aligns himself with postdramatic theatre, which refers to the 'no longer dramatic forms of theatre since the 1970s' generated from starting points other than a stable dramatic text, or that dramatic texts undergo such destabilising treatments that they are no longer at the centre of the work (Lehmann 1). The renowned theatre scholar Hans-Thies Lehmann identifies that some forms of postdramatic theatre are concerned with the exposition of language, the foreignness of the theatre text, and the unnatural process of speaking the theatre text: 'Out of the gaps of language emerges its feared adversary and double: stuttering, failure, accent, flawed pronunciation mark the conflict between body and word' (Lehmann 147). While Cherkaoui is equally interested in foregrounding these gaps of language as are the theatre makers termed postdramatic by Lehmann, there is a strong sense of celebrating these stutters and idiosyncrasies with Cherkaoui. Rather than seeing them as a failure of speaking the text, Cherkaoui regards them as essential non-verbal aspects of oral communication that reveal the speaker's thought processes. Further foregrounding the non-verbal, in relation to Cherkaoui's choreographic treatment of storytelling, he explains: 'So, I like to choreograph body language. [...] Our everyday gestures [...] mean things, so all of us are dancing. All of us are communicating with a form of choreography' (Cherkaoui).

In *zero degrees*, co-choreographer Khan tells the story of his first time visiting Bangladesh and India. While travelling, he discovered that national identity can be determined by something as arbitrary as the colour of a passport. In the story that he tells in unison with Cherkaoui, when the state officials at the border between Bangladesh and India took his passport away from him, Khan realised that without his British passport he no longer has any proof of his identity and panicked. By duplicating the storytelling in a second body, Cherkaoui and Khan reveal the idiosyncrasies in the way the story was originally told. The text is not perfect, but contains hesitations and sentences abandoned midway; however, at the same time it demonstrates richness in movement and gesture stemming from Khan's lifelong experience as a Kathak dancer. The reciting of the story by two people simultaneously is a distancing device that draws attention to the foreignness of the text and the unnatural process of speech alluded to by Lehmann in postdramatic theatre; however, here the distancing is even applied to a non-dramatic, orally based text. Uncannily, because both voices speak at the same time, there is the initial confusion about whose story this is: Khan's or Cherkaoui's? Or do aspects of the story apply to both men? Some scenes of *zero degrees* can be read as Cherkaoui 'trying on' Khan's story to see how it fits in his body. During the creation process, Cherkaoui learnt to perform Khan's grounded, percussive and explosive Kathak-based movement style. The staged work is thus a direct result of this exchange of oral and embodied cultural knowledge. The 'trying on' of Khan's story and movement language is akin to Cherkaoui's wider transcultural search for what is universal in human experience.

Later, in another instalment of Khan's travel story, he encounters a dead body on the train to Calcutta: the man sitting in front of him is not moving anymore and his wife begs the fellow passengers for help. This narrative layer is also visualised choreographically in the separate scene discussed previously, in which Cherkaoui holds hands with the lifeless bodies of the latex dummies and with Khan and reaches out into the audience for help. For a moment, Khan transforms himself into the character of the woman through *abhinaya* (Mitra). Khan's cousin, assuming the role of cultural mediator, prevents him from helping the woman, because the authorities may have mistaken his efforts and Khan would have risked being held responsible for the man's death. Thoughts of death and decay in a place where heat is ever present begin to make Khan feel uncomfortable. He longs to be back at the hotel where he has his conveniences and essential supplies, such as a toilet, bath, a hot shower, television and MTV. Khan's compatibility with his supposed "homeland" seems lost and the contact zone within his own Self exposed (Fig. 3.2).

Fellow performer Cherkaoui again speaks the same story in unison with Khan. However, this time the configuration of the two dancers is different for some parts of the story. While for the initial instalment of the story they begin sitting next to each other facing the audience, in this later scene Cherkaoui lies on his back with his head downstage and his feet upstage, knees pulled up. Khan sits on top of Cherkaoui's knees so that when they speak and gesture in unison, it is as if Cherkaoui represents Khan's reflection in a water surface. Perhaps this becoming aware of his mirror image indicates a greater cultural self-consciousness in Khan as a result of his travelling to the "homeland". Indeed, this is indicative of the auto-ethnographic approach Mitra has identified in Khan's work.

An example of Cherkaoui's own travel stories can be found in the documentary *Rêves de Babel* (2009) about Cherkaoui's life and work. This collaboration between director Don Kent and writer Christian

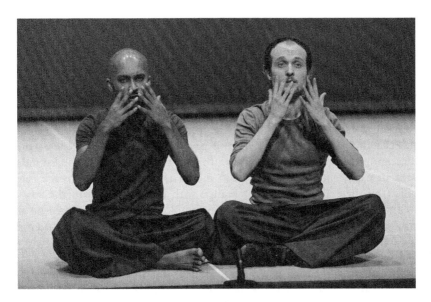

Fig. 3.2 Akram Khan and Sidi Larbi Cherkaoui in *zero degrees* (Photo by Agathe Poupeney)

Dumais-Lyowski was produced by the French Bel Air Média and co-produced by ARTE France. The documentary film-makers followed Cherkaoui as he travelled to four locations, Antwerp, China, Corsica and India, as part of his work to meet people, rehearse together and discuss the productions they were working on at the time. Cherkaoui talks about his work, his identity and his family. The documentary becomes choreographic. The choreography becomes documentary. In *Rêves de Babel*, Cherkaoui tells his own story of travelling to his father's homeland:

> When I was little, I always dreamed of being a musician. When we went to Morocco with my father, he always played Andalusian music in the car, and so, constantly, there was this music which was there, very Arab-Spanish like that, and it made it all... It coloured the whole journey. It took three days of travelling to go down to Morocco, something which we did every year and became a sort of ritual of... to go there. And what I found great, in hindsight, was that it was a journey which made you pass through all these stages: France, very much with its [busy] roads and a certain stress while passing through France; the extreme heat in Spain, the dry coast,

the things we saw, mountains, the dangerous roads on which we drove to get there; then the boats which were like... uh... the feeling of ah finally, water and it... the last little goal in order to arrive to Tangier. So, there was something rather natural about travelling in my childhood.[2]

Storytelling might not seem uncommon in the documentary genre, but Cherkaoui's story would also not seem out of place in one of his own choreographies. He talks about the physical experiences of travelling to his father's homeland as a rite of passage and uses the French word 'descendre' to indicate travelling south, but this word seems to also indicate an experience of descent from modern, stressful, Western life, signified by the representation of France with its busy roads in the story, to the dry heat in Spain, almost unbearable in the days before car air conditioning, to a sense of liberation when he went on the boat to cross the Mediterranean to arrive on what he considered a decisively different continent.

Travelling, it seems, is a significant part of becoming the Other by reconnecting with either the homeland or another site of otherness. Travelling can be a deeply physically transformative experience—the contact zone brought to the surface: vegetarian Willkie experiences a vomit-inducing encounter with goat meat in *Rien de Rien*; in *zero degrees* Khan's eyes play tricks on him whilst trying to determine whether the man opposite him on the train is dead or alive; and in *Rêves de Babel*, Cherkaoui's annual three-day car ride southwards has a profound impact on him as a childhood ritual. These stories present things that were taken for granted in a new light and encourage whoever may be listening to reflect on and evaluate specific aspects of Western society.

In the 1936 essay 'The Storyteller', Walter Benjamin establishes a close connection between travelling and storytelling. The traveller becomes an exotic Other to his listeners, who can shed light on the life beyond their small pre-modern community. Each story contains 'something useful', a 'moral' or 'practical advice', so that the storyteller is considered to have 'counsel' (Benjamin 86). The storytellers in Cherkaoui's works are given a voice, it seems, because they have something interesting to say, something that must be heard particularly to address shortcomings in Western ways of thinking and living. The mixed cultural identity of the performers adds to what Cherkaoui perceives as a richer experience, for example, when travelling, something to be celebrated.

Likewise, in 'Writing Against Culture' feminist anthropologist Lila Abu-Lughod questions what can be gained by including individuals' personal stories in ethnography, arguing for new writing strategies in anthropology. She raises awareness about concerns around the Self/Other distinction in feminist and 'halfie'-ethnography—'halfies' defined as 'people whose national or cultural identity is mixed by virtue of migration, overseas education, or parentage' (Abu-Lughod 466). The difficulty for feminists and 'halfies' when doing ethnography is to accept anthropology's assumption of the fundamental distinction between Self and Other. The boundaries between the Self and studied Other with 'halfie'-ethnographers are not fixed, which renders problematical issues of positionality and objectivity, audience and accountability, and the power inherent in anthropology's Self/Other distinction. Abu-Lughod argues that by their split sense of Self, feminist and 'halfie'-ethnographers challenge anthropology's concept of culture and the tendency that had crept into anthropologists' writing to generalise and to consider cultural difference as fixed and frozen. Therefore, feminist and 'halfie'-ethnographers have created a demand for new writing strategies, because anthropology's traditional 'speaking for' the Other, and thus reinforcing an unequal power-relationship, is no longer desirable. Attention for individual agency and resistance in ethnographic writing acknowledges the divergence between individuals and the negotiating by the individual to position himself in relation to his cultural environment. Abu-Lughod therefore favours writing 'ethnographies of the particular' and devoting attention to individual decision-making, because '(g)eneralization [...] can no longer be regarded as neutral description' (473). However, a space has been opened up for resistance, for example, in minority discourse, where Others can acquire subject-position, represent themselves and show agency to react against oppression, silencing and objectification.

One of Abu-Lughod's central questions is 'Are there ways to write about lives so as to constitute others as less other?' (473). What, then, is the value of bringing the particular into choreography? Similarly to ethnography and anthropology, a shift can be discerned in choreography by artists like Cherkaoui, away from generalisation towards creative employment of cultural position and attention for individual agency and resistance. Performers tell travel stories, sing songs from their childhood, and bring their specific body history to the choreographic language of the work, through their dance traditions or martial arts practices.

Rather than exoticise these cultural elements as Other, which would result in a silencing of the Other, Cherkaoui explores through his choreographies how different cultures can transculturally speak to each other as the stories, songs, and body movement are incorporated in the overarching dramaturgy of the work. 'Halfie'-choreographer Cherkaoui employs his cultural position of a half-Moroccan in Flanders, and those of the performers he chooses to work with, to subvert the surrounding discourse of ethnocentric nationalism, and by doing so, challenges spectators to question their own positionality. In analogy to Abu-Lughod's demand for the new writing strategy of 'ethnographies of the particular', it can be said that Cherkaoui demonstrates what choreographies of the particular would be like. The performers are individuals with a specific cultural position; they are persons, actual people, who employ their cultural position creatively, through their bodies or through their voices, to convey a political message. These dancing bodies are not silent, but eloquent in their particularity. This choreographing—with Abu-Lughod—against culture presents cultural difference beyond the stereotypical, challenging Western hegemony and ethnocentric viewpoints.

The stories in Cherkaoui's choreography, however, function in a very different way from the stories in ethnography. The unison storytelling is an effective choreographic strategy for drawing in the audience in an affective way. Everyday speech is rehearsed, albeit in all its imperfection, as hesitations, pauses, abandoned sentences and quirky manners of speech are meticulously reproduced. The stories are ripped out of the ethnographic context completely, as Cherkaoui tends to include the stories in his works without any of their original contextualisation. It is not made clear where or when the story is set precisely, and by duplicating the story in another body, even who is speaking. Certainty is removed and doubt is introduced, raising more questions than that are answered. There are two performers speaking simultaneously, but whose "voice" is being heard? The spectator flits between intently listening to the story and being distracted by the unison duplication of that story and the choreographically treated body language. Strangely, this choreographic strategy works both to heighten and destabilise perception, as audiences may find themselves incapable of "really" listening to what is said. Abu-Lughod's ethnographies of the particular, by differentiating the Other, work against generalisation and homogenisation; what then is the implication of Cherkaoui's homogenised reproduction of one story in other bodies? This choreographic strategy could be read as a depiction of the generalising mechanism within Western society when confronted with the Other. Anecdotes are taken out of context and come to stand for the whole of the Other culture. The theatrical effect of watching two performers telling the same story simultaneously mirrors the othering mechanism in Western society as a result of inadequate listening. Cherkaoui asks much from the spectator with these unison stories: hearing, listening, seeing, perceiving— perhaps too much. While in anthropology James Clifford argues for a resurgence of the 'ethnographic ear' (12), countering the primarily visualist practices of reading and interpreting by valuing body and sensory perception, Cherkaoui calls upon the spectator's ear to play a more significant role in the process of perception, so that the spectator ultimately becomes more and more physically implicated in the act of watching.

The travel stories in Cherkaoui's works point towards his interest in travel, migration, displacement and destabilised identities, in the sense that these are elements that enrich one's life and need to be celebrated. Cherkaoui, the son of a displaced Moroccan guest labourer in Flanders, seeks to surround himself with performers and collaborators who, like him, have stories to tell of displacement, which is then actively explored through verbal and corporeal storytelling in his work. It is argued that Cherkaoui actively explores and exploits contact zones, especially through working with performers who are aware of the contact zones within the Self due to migration or mixedness, as these tend to reveal cultural difference and friction. Abu-Lughod makes a case for 'halfie'-ethnography by people whose identity is mixed, proposing to favour the writing of 'ethnographies of the particular' that focus on individual decision-making as opposed to generalisation and seemingly neutral description. Likewise, Cherkaoui's exploration of particular cultural elements, such as stories, songs and movement practices, can be read as choreographies of the particular, because he presents cultural difference beyond the stereotypical, challenging Western hegemony and ethnocentrism.

The stories in Cherkaoui's work are given specific choreographic treatment, for example, by duplicating the storytelling in another body in unison in *Rien de Rien* and *zero degrees*. Ripped out of their original context, these stories raise questions about who is speaking and where and when the story is set precisely. The distracting effects of the unison duplication of the gestures accompanying the storytelling may cause the stories and images to linger in the spectator's mind long after the performance, so that the questions raised by the stories can be engaged with as part of the continuous macro dramaturgy of the spectator.

Transculturality Vocalised in Song

Although Khan's central personal narrative in *zero degrees* is immediately apparent, Cherkaoui's narratives and dramaturgical contributions are more veiled and complex, ready to be unpicked by the spectator. Towards the end of the performance, Cherkaoui sits on the floor facing the audience, holding the latex cast of Khan's body on his lap as if he is mourning a loved one, and sings. Khan stands behind the cast of Cherkaoui's body, covering its mouth and drawing his hands away from it, as if he is visualising the sound of a voice resonating into the space. While Khan's lower body remains stable, his legs extended as he shuffles sideways on his feet, his upper body movements become more convulsive and evolve into a violent shaking. There is a clear development in the relationship between Khan's movement and Cherkaoui's song, being similar in dynamics at first and utterly contrasting towards the end. Fragments of the story about the woman pleading for help with the dead body of her husband on the train, visualised by Khan's use of *abhinaya*, echo in my mind.

This theatrical image is full of paradox. Cherkaoui sings the Hebrew song 'Yerushalayim Shel Zahav', which can be translated as 'Jerusalem of Gold', written by Naomi Shemer in 1967 to celebrate Israel's independence. However, on first viewing of *zero* degrees, I did not know this song yet and hence did not realise its full dramaturgic significance. Having identified the language of the song as Hebrew, I was initially content to absorb its musicality and eerie atmosphere, happy to let the scene affect me on a sensorial level. Only afterwards, through speaking with Cherkaoui, did I discover the title of the song, enabling me to dig deeper into its dramaturgic significance. Cherkaoui's Islamic roots and upbringing in a Western country already complicate his cultural identity; the fact that he chooses to sing a song that has become a nationalist Israeli symbol in Hebrew makes for a provocative political statement in the eyes of some spectators (Flanders). Cherkaoui's singing of 'Yerushalayim Shel Zahav' can be seen to invoke the Israeli–Palestinian conflict in *zero degrees*, a dance work that came to fruition during the time of the Second Intifada (2000–2005), which was characterised by bloodshed and illustrative of the diplomatic deadlock in the region. However, he does so without identifying with any particular side and by crossing over into the cultural sphere of the Other.

The first stanza of 'Yerushalayim Shel Zahav' laments the loss of Jerusalem for the Jewish people, whereas in the last stanza the victory is celebrated. The song became a national symbol and unofficial national anthem during the Arab–Israeli War during the 1960s after Israeli troops captured the Old City of Jerusalem and soldiers sang the song to celebrate the liberation of the city (Masalha). However, the song's melody is indebted to the Basque[3] lullaby 'Pello Joxepe'. Although the rhythm has been adapted from an upbeat, bouncy and slightly irregular 3/8 to a clear, steady and regular 3/4 meter, the resemblance of the two melodies is uncanny. 'Pello Joxepe' tends to be improvised with variations to the lyrics. One translation I found indicates that the song is about a man, Peter Joseph, whose wife gives birth to a child that he fears is not his. The song pleads with him not to rush to judgement:

> In this world, Pello Joxepe, we need patience.
> She was your wife, but the child is said to be of another one.
> When the men are out, women spend their time in the forest, amongst brambles.

By suggesting that in their husbands' absence, women are busy foraging rather than cavorting with other men, the song implies that Peter Joseph has got the wrong end of the stick. By being so quick to accuse his wife of infidelity, apparently unjustified, he may have destroyed his marriage and his family at one fell swoop. This cautionary message in the domestic sphere is of interest as a dramaturgical under-layer to Cherkaoui's evocation of the Israeli–Palestinian conflict and, by extension, other wars and conflicts. Perhaps, Cherkaoui is pleading with the global powers to have more patience and not rush to war, particularly when the facts are uncertain. This could be a commentary, for example, on the interventionist foreign policy of the Bush administration leading to the Iraq War at the start of the millennium.

In the final weeks before the premiere of *zero degrees*, articles were published online revealing Shemer's deathbed confession that she had copied the melody of the Basque lullaby. After several years of denying the plagiarism claim, Shemer had confided in a friend that she had used 'Pello Joxepe' unwittingly after hearing someone sing the Basque song in the mid-1960s (Segev). Suggesting that the guilt about concealing this fact, which she had carried for years, may have contributed to her developing cancer, she wrote:

> I consider the entire affair a regrettable work accident - so regrettable that it may be the reason for me taking ill. [...] My only comfort is that I tell myself that perhaps it is a tune of the Anusim [Spanish or Portuguese Jews who were forced to convert and kept Jewish practices in secret] and all I did was restore past glory. (Shemer qtd. in Segev)

This is an interesting possibility, which, if this is the indeed the case, means that the transculturality of this song would then have gone full circle. When Cherkaoui performs the Hebrew song in *zero degrees*, he abandons the 3/4 meter of Shemer's song, occasionally using the entire duration of his exhalation for certain syllables. The song becomes extremely protracted and eerie, working on the spectator on an affective level, particularly in its combination with the convulsive choreography performed by Khan. This may prompt spectators to question what the song is and where it comes from, thus exposing its unexpected origins. This continuous macro-dramaturgical engagement with certain elements from *zero degrees* established with confidence that Cherkaoui's choreographic negotiations of geopolitical critique and national identity are grounded in a strong awareness of the transcultural permeability of culture, and an understanding of identity as kaleidoscopic, fragmented, composite and continually shifting and realigned.

Cherkaoui is eager to point out in conversation that many of the cultural, nationalistic symbols that are considered to be authentic and pure actually originate from different cultures and are not as unambiguous as people assume them to be. The circles of possible cultural influence, from Basque onto Israeli song and from oppressed Jews onto Basque folk culture, seem to reverberate endlessly in this single theatrical image and the sound waves produced by Cherkaoui's voice. This subsequent questioning of elements from the work after the performance moment forms part of the continuous macro-dramaturgical work the spectator completes in response to Cherkaoui's work. By unveiling this disorderly cross-pollination of cultures, Cherkaoui dismantles the claim for purity of origins when he performs this song.

'Pello Joxepe' is a folk song, orally transmitted and often improvised with different versions of the lyrics, whereas Shemer has appropriated its melody for her song which turned into a nationalistic symbol. Through 'Pello Joxepe's' very absence, Cherkaoui may hence be pointing at the power imbalances between written and oral cultures. Orally transmitted cultural material is not subject to ownership or copyright; instead, it is owned collectively and subtly yet continuously transformed through encounters with cultural others. Similar to the stories he includes, orally transmitted songs, like 'Pello Joxepe' and those from the Mediterranean region in other works, are the bearers of pre-modern transculturality.

Ultimately, Cherkaoui's aim with this theatrical image is to demonstrate a pluralistic approach to the complex issue of the Israeli–Palestinian conflict, countering one-sided and ethnocentric views. During an informal conversation in December 2008, Cherkaoui explained that in his opinion, there is no longer a straightforward victim and/or aggressor in this situation. With this awareness that social concepts such as that of the nation are constructed and often constricting, nationalistic and ethnocentric ideas are difficult to retain. Instead, Cherkaoui proposes a flexible approach to such complex political issues as the Israeli–Palestinian conflict, utilising multiple viewpoints simultaneously, emphasising the transcultural networks that connect cultures and refusing a dogmatic, singular stance.

Cherkaoui's viewpoint seems to be based on the cosmopolitan idea that all human beings belong to the same community and have responsibilities of justice and hospitality towards each other beyond state boundaries. Cherkaoui's circle of artistic collaborators, and by extension his choreographic work, exemplifies this kind of cosmopolitan openness to different cultures, languages, dance idioms, musicalities, approaches and ideas. He, the company, and the work itself, travel the world in a cosmopolitan way, either as part of creation or performance. In certain strands of cosmopolitanism, cultures, too, are regarded to be unfixed entities, constantly influenced by, and influencing, other cultures (Scheffler; Appiah). '[A]ll cultures simply *are* cosmopolitan mixtures, evolving in interaction with other cultures, so that we are all "naturally" hybrid and it is purification that is taught and imposed' (Rao 20).

In line with Maalouf, this cosmopolitan emphasis on the permeability of culture, and indeed transculturality, challenges an exaggerated sense of national identity and therefore nationalist discourses. Cherkaoui's choreographic negotiations of the nation as construct favour a kaleidoscopic approach to identity, in which different and intersecting aspects of identity are balanced. In Maalouf's writing on identity as composite and characterised by multiplicity, Cherkaoui found affirmation of his kaleidoscopic approach to identity as fragmented, ever-shifting and constantly realigned and reoriented. For Cherkaoui, national identity is but one aspect of identity and he is cautious of allowing it to overpower the other dimensions of identity.

Influenced by cosmopolitanism, he is interested in what people have in common, rather than that what sets them apart, and entertains the idea that dance, rhythm and movement play a key role in that, while his utopian aim is to improve understanding between people from different cultures (Olaerts). Through his creative process of collaboration and imitation, both in choreographic and in gestural movement languages, as well as speech and song, Cherkaoui is proposing this process of choreographically becoming the Other as a possible answer to deadlock, impasse, war even. The transformation of the self into the Other—a present Other in his co-performer Khan or an absent Other as in the Israeli soldiers singing 'Yerushalayim Shel Zahav'—is an important exercise for him not to get stuck in his own movement language, his own language and musicality, and hence by extension his own identity and world view. Each person's understanding of the world is necessarily limited. Cherkaoui himself has characterised his approach as that of a chameleon, in an interview with Cools: 'I trust more and more the flexibility of my own body to take on different shapes and colors like a chameleon' (60). Without wanting to institute a Cartesian body-mind split, this readiness to transform his body also extends to the flexibility of his mind, or body-mind, the way he perceives the world.

These activities of continuously engaging with the Other, through attentive listening and imitation for the performers in the work, but also through the attentive watching and dramaturgical engagement which the spectator is invited to do, stand for the larger hermeneutic project of understanding the world in all its complexities. Even though understanding alone cannot move conflict out of deadlock, awareness of paradox and complexity and acknowledgement of the viewpoint of the Other can be considered the first step towards resolution.

ETHNOGRAPHY AND THE LIMITS OF TRANSCULTURALISM

The exploration of what is shared in common with others and of transformation, momentarily becoming the Other through choreographic movement, is also at the heart of *Sutra*. The Sadler's Wells production, based on Cherkaoui's visit to and subsequent collaborative work with the monks of the Shaolin Temple in Dengfeng county in the Henan province in China, celebrated its tenth anniversary touring season in the spring of 2018. Cherkaoui was pursuing a childhood fascination with Kung Fu, which he encountered through the martial arts films of Bruce Lee.

The groundwork for his own physical exploration of Kung Fu was already laid during the creation of *zero degrees*, which features a shadow-boxing scene with Khan. Over time, Cherkaoui also became drawn towards 'the philosophy underpinning the form – the idea that all living creatures are part of a universal energy and that the movements of kung fu [sic] are a means of channelling that force' (Mackrell). Without equating the two ways of thinking, it is possible to see a tentative connection between the universality at the heart of Chan Buddhism and Cherkaoui's commitment to transcultural exploration, intent on what binds people and cultures together rather than what sets them apart. Although in some respects Cherkaoui and the Chinese monks of the Shaolin Temple could not be more different from one another—their daily lives were vastly dissimilar and they needed a translator to communicate—Cherkaoui was eager to explain that he sees significant similarities between himself and the monks as well:

> I went [to the Shaolin temple] in May last year and I had an incredible experience. It was only for five days but I really felt suddenly home: I felt home. It has to do with very simple things. I've been a vegetarian for 17 years, I never drink, I never smoke – I don't do any of those things that are very common in my culture. In Belgian culture we drink beer all the time and in Arab culture they smoke and eat meat. So in my daily life I always felt a little bit like an alien – and there I am in the temple where suddenly vegetarian food is the norm – and they drink tea and respect life. And also they're very disciplined with their bodies. (Cherkaoui qtd. in Londondance)

Returning to the concept of kaleidoscopic identity introduced at the start of the book, the choreographer adds even more aspects to his selfhood here: vegetarianism and sobriety. He therefore steers the debate away again from national identity, race and religion, the aspects of identity with which the populist radical right is most concerned. By emphasising his own otherness through his personal life choices, Cherkaoui also attempts to reverse the othering, exoticising mechanisms Western audiences tend to employ in their encounters with Chinese performing troupes. However, this study of *Sutra* will evaluate the limits of Cherkaoui's transcultural creative process visible in the choreographic aesthetic of the work when the main mode of operation was ultimately one of ethnography. Cherkaoui has choreographed himself into the work as an outsider, an observer, a 'wannabe' Kung Fu warrior even. Further exploring postcolonial critiques of ethnography, this section asks what the dramaturgical potential is of this aesthetic exposing of the limits of transculturalism through Cherkaoui's visualising of the ethnographic nature of his creative inquiry in the choreography of *Sutra* itself (Fig. 3.3).

Sutra was Cherkaoui's second collaboration with visual artist Gormley, after *zero degrees* and before *Babel*$^{(words)}$ (co-choreographed with Damien Jalet, 2010); *zero degrees* and *Sutra* hence are the first and second part of a different trilogy of Cherkaoui-Gormley collaborations. Cherkaoui's other key creative partners for *Sutra* include the Polish composer Szymon Brzóska, dramaturges Lou Cope and An-Marie Lambrechts, choreography assistants Ali Ben Lotfi Thabet (who had performed in *Tempus Fugit*), Satoshi Kudo and Damien Fournier (who had both performed in *Myth*) and Jalet. Thabet, Kudo and Fournier have all performed the role Cherkaoui created for himself when *Sutra* is on tour, thereby freeing the choreographer up to undertake other projects rather than perform each and every show. Dance scholar Sabine Sörgel offers

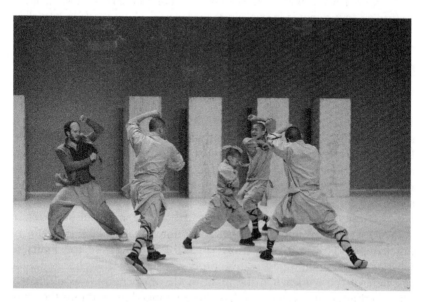

Fig. 3.3 *Sutra* (Photo by Agathe Poupeney)

a detailed analysis of the work, enriched by research of the philosophical principles and practices of Kung Fu. She frames *Sutra* as a 'danced investigation of Chan-mind [the Buddhist precepts underpinning Kung Fu] through the eyes of the Western choreographer' (Sörgel 188). My responses to the work in this chapter seek to analyse selected aspects in terms of their significance from the broader dramaturgical strategies Cherkaoui developed in his oeuvre at the time, most notably transculturality and the macro-dramaturgical relationship between the work and the spectator, in other words the ways in which theatre begins to fulfil its social function.

In terms of its general structure, *Sutra* shows a group of 18 warrior monks, all aged around 20 or 21 and all dressed the same in a traditional Kung Fu training outfit and footwear initially and later wearing a modern suit and T-shirt. There is also a child on stage, the ten-year-old Shi Yandong, nicknamed 'Dong Dong', who is a novice at the temple. Then there is Cherkaoui, whose clothes are slightly different from the monks': he wears a button-down shirt with the traditional trousers, along with a suit jacket and white trainers, making him stand out as a Westerner. At times, the group of monks perform Kung Fu movements in unison, or in a near-unison rapid canon that visualises the speed of their actions, while Cherkaoui looks from the side lines but does not join in. The movement sequences the monks perform are slow and contemplative on a few occasions and explosive and spectacular on others, employing staffs and swords. Cherkaoui dances a number of solos, which are melancholic, yet playful, reminiscent of the mime Marcel Marceau. For example, he pretends to go down some stairs in a wooden box where there are no stairs. He demonstrates his personal movement preferences for continuous, circular movements of the limbs and contortionism. Cherkaoui also dances a number of duets with Dong Dong, the child novice, with whom it seems he was able to establish a special rapport in the creative process through play. They dance inside a wooden box as if they are caught inside and are trying to either escape or accept their fate.

The movements performed by the group of monks only infrequently diverge from the Kung Fu practice in which they are trained. In a brief solo, one of the monks expands his movements by tracing his index finger through the space, a sequence which may have been derived from the type of improvisation task Cherkaoui tended to employ for some of his other works such as *Rien de Rien* or *Foi*, perhaps in an attempt to explore different creative processes with the monks and make the

Kung Fu movements more 'choreographic'. When the monks perform solo rather than unison, there are moments of greater choreographic integration. Each of the monks performs a short sequence of movement which represents the energy of a certain animal, including a cat, monkey or scorpion. Here, Cherkaoui does join in and performs movements of his own that resemble those of a scorpion, with both hands on the floor, his torso kept low and one leg lifted up behind like the scorpion's tail. His scorpion engages in a choreographic dialogue with the monks' animals. These interactions are rare and show Cherkaoui relishing the moments when his personal movement vocabulary, typified by fluid floorwork and flexibility, intersects with the movement material of the monks. There is one scene in which all the monks sit cross-legged on top of wooden boxes and perform an extended movement sequence derived from sign language, which Cherkaoui or one of his assistants, likely to have been Fournier, must have taught them. The DVD recording reveals insecurity on some of the monks' faces as they tentatively explore new movements. It is a rare occasion of the monks moving closer to Cherkaoui and his choreographic practice, if the entire *Sutra* project should not already be interpreted as such. Overall, the choreographic balance in *Sutra* swings to a visual distinction between the relatively homogeneous group of monks and Dong Dong and Cherkaoui as outsiders, as Others, even as Dong Dong matures during the work into becoming more and more integrated with the monks. This otherness is further reinforced through the work's visual design, which helps to articulate the dramaturgical approach in this work.

Gormley's design for *Sutra* consists of a set of man-size wooden boxes, open on one side like coffins and three times as high as they are wide. These dimensions mean that the boxes can easily be stacked in different configurations and used as building blocks, like a 'mobile architecture' (Sörgel 187). Throughout the work, the meanings these boxes take on constantly shift and transform depending on their orientation or configuration: bunk-beds, shipping containers, sentry boxes, a maze, a rabbit hutch, a lotus flower opening, dominoes, tortoise shells, a vessel, a temple arch. Downstage right, there is a small-scale model of the boxes, which Cherkaoui and Dong Dong manipulate between them, sometimes instigating the configurations of the life-size boxes on the rest of the stage, sometimes merely paralleling their movements and sometimes catching up (Fig. 3.4).

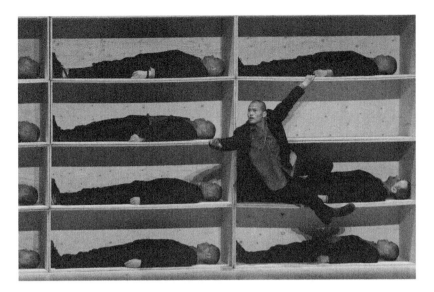

Fig. 3.4   *Sutra* (Photo by Agathe Poupeney)

There is one box made of aluminium, predominantly occupied by Cherkaoui. Aesthetically, it stands out as an anomaly against the unclad wood colour of the other boxes. Gormley explains that: 'Larbi wanted his aluminium box, and it was sweet how much he wanted it. So we made one. ... I wasn't sure whether it deserved to be there; it rather undermines the others' (Duguid). Cherkaoui's dramaturgical drive for his box to look distinctive, against the wishes of Gormley and his overall design, is indicative of his insistence that he is an outsider in the work and was an outsider during the creative process. One might wonder why Cherkaoui choreographed himself into the work in the first place. He might have opted to choreograph a work just for the monks and leave himself as choreographer invisible from the staged work. Or he might have crafted his own role in the work on a par with the monks, wearing the same costumes, occupying an identical wooden box and performing the same movements. Neither of those options, however, would have enabled Cherkaoui to draw attention to the process of ethnography as translation between cultures. In the previous sections, we have already explored some postcolonial critiques of ethnography, though the work of Abu-Lughod. Robin Patric Clair explains that ethnography, as the study of the Other, is founded on the master discourse of European imperialism and hence even asks 'whether the concept *postcolonial ethnography* should be considered an oxymoron' (19). With *Sutra*, Cherkaoui reveals a fascination with ethnography as a mode of cultural dialogue and translation, but equally a critical awareness of the postcolonial limits of ethnography. However, for all the critiques, Cherkaoui is not ready to outright reject ethnography and sticks with it as a choreographic mode in *Sutra*.

Sörgel connects the 'life-affirming spiritualism' in Cherkaoui's choreographic work and that of others to 'an affective mediation of dance's political claim to agency and autonomy', which is predicated on 'cross-cultural collaboration and diplomacy across national boundaries' (198). Even if, in *Sutra*, Cherkaoui must resort to revealing the ethnographic nature of his creative inquiry as a dramaturgical strategy because this work's creative process did not reach the far-reaching transculturalism that permeates other works such as *zero degrees*, he still employed the transcultural question of what is shared between cultures as a starting point. With his visit to the Shaolin Temple, Cherkaoui was pursuing his own growth and transformation, but in the choreographic work that resulted from that process he is careful to show the limits of this transformation. At best, he was able to move closer to this community at the Shaolin Temple, to learn from the monks and learn about himself as a result; however, he was not able to begin to lift the distinction between himself and 'them'. In his choreography, Cherkaoui reflected these limitations rather than glossing over them or glorifying his encounter.

Notes

1. The notion of the suspension of disbelief has been further developed from its origins in relation to Romantic poetry within animation studies discourses (Dobson, Honess Roe, Ratelle & Ruddell).
2. Translation by the author of: 'Quand j'étais petit, je rêvais toujours d'être musicien. Quand on allait en Maroc avec mon père, il mettait toujours de la musique Andalous dans la voiture, et donc, constamment, on avait ce musique qui était là, très Arabe-Espagnol comme ça, et ça faisait toute une… ça colorait tout le voyage. C'étaient trois jours de voyage pour descendre vers le Maroc, quelque chose qu'on faisait tous les ans et ça devenait un sort de rituel de… pour y aller. Et ce que je trouvais bien, avec le recul, c'était que c'était un voyage qui se faisait passer par tous les

stades: la France, tellement avec les chemins et un certain stress en passant la France; la chaleur en Espagne extrême, le côté sèche, les choses qu'on voyait, les montagnes, les chemins dangereuses sur lesquelles on roulait pour y arriver; puis les bateaux qui étaient comme... euh... le sentiment de ah enfin, l'eau et le... dernier petit bout pour arriver en Tanger. Donc il y avait quelque chose d'assez naturelle dans mon enfance de voyage'.

3. The construction of Basque national identity and consequent claims to autonomy should be historically located in the project of modernity (Díaz Noci). Arguably, this could be seen to apply to the Flemish nationalist and Zionist movements too. The autonomy claims of these different groups also seem to resonate with Maalouf's concept that when a certain aspect of people's identity is threatened, such as their Flemishness, or Basqueness or Jewishness, this aspect often becomes more important than other aspects of their composite identity and may mobilise them into defensive action.

BIBLIOGRAPHY

Abu-Lughod, Lila. 'Writing Against Culture'. 1991. *Anthropology in Theory: Issues in Epistemology.* Ed. Moore, Henrietta L. & Sanders, Todd. Malden, MA: Blackwell, 2005. 466–479. Print.

Appiah, Kwame Anthony. *Cosmopolitanism: Ethics in a World of Strangers.* New York: W. W. Norton, 2006. Print.

Benjamin, Walter. *Illuminations.* New York: Schocken Books, 1968. Print.

Bhabha, Homi K. 'Culture's In-Between'. *Questions of Cultural Identity.* Ed. Gay, Paul de & Hall, Stuart. London: Sage, 1996. 53–60. Print.

Bond, Lucy & Rapson, Jessica. Eds. *The Transcultural Turn: Interrogating Memory Between and Beyond Borders.* Berlin: Walter de Gruyter, 2014. Print.

Clair, Robin Patric. 'The Changing Story of Ethnography'. *Expressions of Ethnography: Novel Approaches to Qualitative Methods.* Ed. Clair, Robin Patric. 2003. Web. Accessed: 9 August 2018. <https://www.sunypress.edu/pdf/60804.pdf>.

Clifford, James & Marcus, George E. *Writing Culture: The Poetics and Politics of Ethnography.* Berkeley, CA: University of California Press, 1986. Print.

Cools, Guy. *In-Between Dance Cultures: On the Migratory Artistic Identity of Sidi Larbi Cherkaoui and Akram Khan.* Antennae Series. Amsterdam: Valiz, 2015. Print.

Díaz Noci, Javier. 'The Creation of the Basque Identity Through Cultural Symbols in Modern Times'. *Ehu.es.* 1999. Web. Accessed: 20 September 2009. <http://www.ehu.es/diaz-noci/Conf/C17.pdf>.

Dobson, Nichola; Honess Roe, Annabelle; Ratell, Amy & Ruddell, Caroline. Eds. *The Animation Studies Reader.* London: Bloomsbury Academic, 2018. Print.

Duguid, Hannah. 'A Box of Delights: Antony Gormley's "Sutra"'. *The Independent*. 2008. Web. Accessed: 25 July 2018. <https://www.independent.co.uk/arts-entertainment/art/features/a-box-of-delights-antony-gormleys-sutra-831379.html>.

Fensham, Rachel & Kelada, Odette. 'Dancing the Transcultural Across the South'. *Journal of Intercultural Studies*. 33.4. (2012): 363–373. Print.

Flanders, Judith. 'Zero Degrees Is a True Meeting of Equals'. *Guardian Unlimited*. 2007. Web. Accessed: 9 November 2007. <http://blogs.guardian.co.uk/theatre/2007/10/zero_degrees_is_a_true_meeting.html>.

Gilbert, Jenny. 'Dunas, Sadler's Wells, London: The Odd Couple Do a Sand Dance'. *The Independent*. 2011. Web. Accessed: 6 August 2018. <https://www.independent.co.uk/arts-entertainment/theatre-dance/reviews/dunas-sadlers-wells-london-2280716.html>.

Jennings, Luke. 'Dunas; May—Review'. *The Guardian*. 2011. Web. Accessed: 4 August 2018. <https://www.theguardian.com/stage/2011/may/08/dunas-sadlers-wells-review>.

Khoury, Krystel. 'Un arbre aux possibilités multiples: Le traitement de la main dans le travail chorégraphique de Sidi Larbi Cherkaoui'. *Des mains modernes: Cinéma, danse, photographie, théâtre*. Ed. André, Emmanuelle; Palazzolo, Claudia & Siety, Emmanuel. Paris: L'Harmattan, 2008. 14–26. Print.

Lehmann, Hans-Thies. (trans. Karen Juers-Munby) *Postdramatic Theatre*. London: Routledge, 2006. Print.

Londondance. 'Interview: Sidi Larbi Cherkaoui Q&A'. 2008. Web. Accessed: 25 July 2018. <http://londondance.com/articles/interviews/sidi-larbi-cherkaoui-qanda/>.

Maalouf, Amin. *In the Name of Identity: Violence and the Need to Belong*. New York: Random House, 2000. Print.

Mackrell, Judith. 'Sutra.' *The Guardian*. 2008. Web. Accessed: 25 July 2018. <https://www.theguardian.com/stage/2008/may/30/dance>.

Masalha, Nur. *The Bible and Zionism: Invented Traditions, Archaeology and Postcolonialism in Palestine-Israel*. London: Zed Books, 2007. Print.

Mitra, Royona. *Akram Khan: Dancing New Interculturalism*. New World Choreographies Series. London: Palgrave Macmillan. 2015. Print.

Morin, Justin. *Sidi Larbi Cherkaoui: Pèlerinage Sur Soi*. Arles: Actes Sud, 2006. Print.

Olaerts, An. 'Marokkaan uit Hoboken én Choreograaf van het Jaar'. *Vacature*. 31 October 2008. 14–17. Print.

Pratt, Marie Louise. *Imperial Eyes: Travel Writing and Transculturation*. 2nd Ed. London: Routledge, 2007. Print.

Rao, Rahul. 'Postcolonial Cosmopolitanism: Between Home and the World'. D.Phil. Thesis, Politics and International Relations, University of Oxford. 2007. Web. Accessed: 15 April 2009. <http://ora.ouls.ox.ac.uk/objects/uuid:6eb91e22-9563-49a2-be2b-402a4edd99b5>.

Scheffler, Samuel. *Boundaries and Allegiances: Problems of Justice and Responsibility in Liberal Thought*. Oxford: Oxford University Press, 2001. Print.

Segev, Tom. 'Naomi Shemer Lifted Jerusalem of Gold Melody from Basque Folk Song'. *Haaretz*. 2005. Web. Accessed: 19 October 2008. <http://www.haaretz.com/naomi-shemer-lifted-jerusalem-of-gold-melody-from-basque-folk-song-1.157828>.

Sörgel, Sabine. *Dance and the Body in Western Theatre: 1948 to the Present*. London: Red Globe Press, 2015. Print.

Tutek, Hrovje. 'Limits to Transculturality: A Book Review Article of New Work by Kimmich and Schahadat and Juvan'. *CLCWeb: Comparative Literature and Culture*. 15.5. (2013). Web. Accessed: 18 August 2017. <http://docs.lib.purdue.edu/cgi/viewcontent.cgi?article=2352&context=clcweb>.

Van Kerkhoven, Marianne. 'Looking Without Pencil in the Hand'. *Theaterschrift*. 5–6. (1994): 140–148. Print.

Welsch, Wolfgang. 'Transculturality—The Puzzling Form of Cultures Today'. *Spaces of Culture: City, Nation, World*. Ed. Featherstone, Mike & Lash, Scott. London: Sage, 1999. 194–213. Print.

Woolf, Diana. 'Maker of the Month/Kei Ito'. *Ideas in the Making*. 2010. Web. Accessed: 8 August 2018. <http://www.themaking.org.uk/Content/makers/2010/01/kei_ito.html>.

Multimedia Sources

Pello Joxepe. 'Traditional Basque Song Performed by Paco Ibañez'. 2008. Song. Accessed: 6 June 2008. <http://www.youtube.com/watch?v=ttuRcl1dK1M>.

Rêves de Babel/Dreams of Babel. Created by Sidi Larbi Cherkaoui. Directed by Don Kent. BelAir Media. 2010. DVD.

Sutra. Choreographed by Sidi Larbi Cherkaoui. Sadler's Wells. Axiom Films. 2008. DVD.

Yerushalayim Shel Zahav. Written and Performed by Naomi Shemer. 1967. Song.

Zero Degrees. Co-choreographed by Sidi Larbi Cherkaoui and Akram Khan. Sadler's Wells. Axiom Films. 2008. DVD.

Zéro Degré: L'Infini. Created by Gilles Delmas. Lardux Films. 2006. DVD.

Thematic Explorations of Religion in *Foi* and *Apocrifu*

Cherkaoui's privileging of orality and storytelling indicates a distrust of the written word and the hegemony of Western history. This idea will be elaborated further in this chapter, focusing on his distrust of religious fundamentalist discourse, which elevates religious texts as 'the Word of God' as a key macro-dramaturgical focus. Cherkaoui actively explores religious themes in many of his works. Cherkaoui's earliest work to explicitly use religion as a main theme was *Foi* (2003). 'Foi' can be translated from the French as 'belief'. The work included Christian imagery of the suffering Christ and the Pietà, as well as angels and halos. Orally transmitted religious music from the Mediterranean region was juxtaposed to both sacred and secular music from the Ars Nova period, highlighting another of Cherkaoui's central creative explorations since *Rien de Rien* (2000). After *Foi, Tempus Fugit* (2004) contained scenes of the ritual washing of hands and faces, and a veiled woman performing an agonised solo while inhaling and exhaling through a harmonica, which can be seen to represent her voice being silenced by Islam. *Myth* (2007) continued to excavate religious symbols, most prominently that of the cross, in the wider context of myth and Jungian psychoanalysis. *Apocrifu* (2007), however, is again, like *Foi*, primarily focused on the immediate choreographic exploration of religion.

From a biographical point of view, it is significant to pause and note again that Cherkaoui grew up in a multi-religious family, his father being Muslim and his mother Catholic. As a boy, he attended Qur'an school under the influence of his father, while his main primary and secondary

© The Author(s) 2019   103
L. Uytterhoeven, *Sidi Larbi Cherkaoui*, New World Choreographies,
https://doi.org/10.1007/978-3-030-27816-8_4

education took place in the secular sector, as evidenced by a reference he made to 'morality studies', the secular alternative to 'religious studies' in the curriculum in primary and secondary education in Flanders. Through his Flemish mother and the larger context of growing up in the predominantly Catholic Flanders of the late twentieth century, Cherkaoui also became permeated with Catholic ideas and imagery. The rise of the populist radical right in Flanders since the 1980s, especially in Antwerp where he grew up, had a significant impact on him. Part of this extreme right discourse is infused with xenophobic and Islamophobic thoughts. Therefore, during Cherkaoui's youth, religion was continuously contested and never straightforward or unquestioned, which may have contributed to his critical stance towards religious fundamentalism.

Fundamentalism became an acute global issue after the terrorist attacks in the USA on 11 September 2001. Many of Cherkaoui's key works gathered in this book for analysis were created in the wake of the 2001 terrorist attacks and the ensuing War on Terror in Iraq and Afghanistan and can be seen to address aspects of the debates about religious fundamentalism. The Islamic studies scholar Malise Ruthven, however, clarifies that religious fundamentalism has been at the root of major conflicts since the end of the Cold War in the late 1980s. Although often intertwined with issues of ethnicity and nationalism, religion has become a crucial aspect of identity for many and 'seems to have replaced the old ideologies of Marxist-Leninism, national socialism, anti-colonialism as the principal challenge to the world order based on the hegemonic power of the liberal capitalist West' (Ruthven 3–4). This chapter will discuss Cherkaoui's thematic exploration of religion in *Foi* and *Apocrifu* in the light of transreligious theological perspectives, which he mobilises creatively and dramaturgically to undermine religious fundamentalism. With regard to *Apocrifu*, the discussion in this chapter focuses on his choreographic representation of religious texts as man-made and intertexual, distrusting the elevation of the religious written word. Hence, this choreographic strategy may be understood to be parallel to Cherkaoui's challenging of written history through the foregrounding of storytelling and orality, explored in the previous chapter. This analysis of *Apocrifu* will be set within a broader historical context by highlighting events that dominated the news in the Western world since the late 1980s, which bring to the fore arguments related to fundamentalism.

Transreligious Theology

Cherkaoui's continued critical exploration of religion is at heart transreligious. Emerging from comparative theology and interreligious studies, transreligious theological discourse is predicated on the principle of dialogue and transformative processes (Faber). Outward-facing, interreligious dialogue gives rise to inward, transformative processes, or 'movements' (Faber 74), so that its goal is not one of comparison, but deepening understanding. In this way, it 'gives rise to new theological thoughts and theories' (Tracy qtd. in Faber 74). Theological discourses, like cultures in transcultural modes of thinking, are hence seen not as closed and fixed, but porous and open to transformation and development. The transreligious endeavour is described as a 'theology without walls [...] not in thrall to specific sacred texts, not limited to specific confessional documents, and not on behalf of concrete religious traditions' (Wildman 243). This transreligious perspective destabilises the very grounds on which religious fundamentalism is balanced.

The theologian and scholar of world religions John J. Thatamanil advocates passionately for transreligious theology on the grounds that it offers a set of resources with which to create integrated meanings from the diversity, hybridity and multiplicities in the globalised world. Transreligious theology is defined as 'a mode of truth seeking enquiry that draws upon the resources of more than one tradition' (Thatamanil 355). Not necessarily conducted from a point of view of belonging to a particular religious tradition, from which one crosses over to another and then returns to one's own, transreligious theology instead presupposes that 'other more complex patterns of affiliation or non-affiliation' are possible, including, like in Cherkaoui's case, no direct religious affiliation at all (Thatamanil 355). Hence, transreligious theology is disconnected from religious identity. What sets this mode of thinking apart from conventional comparative theology is that the transreligious 'encounter with the other is a subject to subject relation—persons from other traditions are understood to be fellow inquirers into the truth about ultimate matters' (Thatamanil 356). From a place of vulnerability, the transreligious theologian engages with the interpretive schemes and therapeutic regimens of other religious traditions, open to learning from what others have come to know. This approach is at the heart of Cherkaoui's transcultural creative process that resists the colonial echoes of ethnography, discussed in the previous chapter in relation to *zero degrees* and *Sutra*.

Cherkaoui transforms himself into the Other through the practicing of their movement practices for the purpose of gaining a deeper understanding of life, culture and humanity as an ultimate truth, not as a way of acquiring knowledge to contain and dominate the Other. Hence, Cherkaoui's choreographic and dramaturgic practice, as far as the exploration of religious traditions is concerned, is not only transcultural but also transreligious.

FOI AS A TRANSRELIGIOUS CREATIVE INQUIRY

Foi, performed by Les Ballets C. de la B. and Flemish ensemble Capilla Flamenca, led by Dirk Snellings, premiered in Ghent, Belgium, on 18 March 2003. During the initial generative phases of the creative process for *Foi*, Cherkaoui used the question 'What do you believe in?' as a starting point, inviting the international group of co-creating performers to give their own meanings to the term 'belief'. Stories of family and close human connections emerged in parallel to the performers' personal experiences of religion and its limits.

Foi begins with an image that depicts the world after a catastrophe, as people's bodies and furniture are scattered across the stage floor. Soon, it becomes clear that there are some survivors. The protagonists, Christine Leboutte, Joanna Dudley, Ulrika Kinn Svensson and Darryl E. Woods, are dressed in bright red, green or blue pedestrian clothes, such as suits, dresses and shoes. In an interview early on in my research process in 2004, Cherkaoui explained that this group represents the mortals on earth. They work within the lowest level of the stage design, the stage floor, bordered between two menacing and impenetrable grey walls. The protagonists are trying to come to terms with their memories of those they lost, as well as trying to find a way to continue with their lives. Cherkaoui has hence pitched his transreligious exploration of belief at the exact moment when a person's belief may be tested: at the time of bereavement and catastrophe. His investigation tests what people can and do fall back on in moments of crisis. The protagonists are influenced and manipulated by angel-like creatures, Lisbeth Gruwez (whose role was later danced by Alexandra Gilbert from January 2004 onwards), Jalet, Nam Jin Kim, Laura Neyskens, Erna Ómarsdóttir, Nicolas Vladyslav and Marc Wagemans. The angels share the stage floor with the mortals and wear pale-coloured trousers and a shirt or dress, and generally move barefoot. The group referred to by Cherkaoui as 'the gods', is performed by the seven musicians of Capilla Flamenca. They witness the events happening on the stage floor from above, from a gallery high up in the left wall, looking through three windows that resemble a triptych painting. They are dressed in beige suits. Cherkaoui explains that

> the number three dominates: the Holy Trinity, three religions, three chapters [a temporal structure to the performance, divided by a black-out], three windows acting as a triptych, and a triangular stage created by two high walls. The creation of the dance sequences often also takes place in groups of three, forming a circular movement, a perpetuum mobile. Three letters also form the name of the performance, *Foi*. (Cherkaoui in Capilla Flamenca 9)

Initially, the protagonists are scattered, lying on the floor in haphazard positions among various items of furniture and covered in a thick layer of dust and debris. A woman with short dark hair (Dudley), dressed in a bright green skirt suit, gets up and announces a list of flights and flight numbers that have been cancelled into a public address (PA) system, which renders the sound of her voice metallic and emotionally detached. The angels enter the space, whispering, and position themselves close to the various protagonists. A middle-aged woman with long hair draped around her face (Leboutte), holds up an A4-sized photo of a young man's face—who, it will later be suggested, represents her dead son (Jalet). Then, an elderly female character, played by the African American actor and dancer Woods in drag, wakes and rises with her fake buttocks high up in the air, groaning and moaning. She looks around the stage, acknowledging the other people with quotes from the Bible. Originally from Alabama, Woods speaks with an American accent from the Southern states. The exaggeration of the extreme high and low intonation specifically has a comical effect. Svensson is the last protagonist to be introduced; she plays a weather lady. The angels manipulate the protagonists into a variety of pedestrian actions. While two angels twirl around her and prod her with various body parts, Dudley is moved by them into a shrug of the shoulders, waving some hair out of her face, exaggerated breathing, scratching her face, looking around and some quiet, discrete crying. Leboutte asks the other protagonists: 'Have you seen my son?' in multiple languages. They ignore her. Svensson is tickled by her angels, causing her to laugh hysterically.

Later, Neyskens initiates a frantic Flamenco-inspired tap dance, which evolves into an earthquake, as all the performers are shaking themselves and the furniture vigorously. Vladyslav rises into a handstand centre stage, which leads him to perform a virtuosic solo based on circular, never-ending movements as he moves on and across the floor, performing jumps, twists and reaches. Capilla Flamenca sing 'Gloria: Missa Notre Dame', which is characterised by beautiful harmonies and extended *melismata*. The spectacular, protracted 'Amen' is visualised by another handstand by Vladyslav, who sustains this position for a long while.

The earthquake resumes and there are numerous loud screams, which culminate in a groaning Woods seemingly giving birth to a naked, yet full-grown, Vladyslav. Woods quotes Steve Urkel, a character from the American 1990s sitcom *Family Matters*, asking 'Did I do that?' while he points at Vladyslav, and then sings a few lines of the popular song 'Baby Love' (1964). Moments later, Svensson and Vladyslav, who is now clad in a dark suit, engage in a nervous flirty conversation; however, she speaks English and he speaks French. They seem to misunderstand each other and perform a clumsy body language. They bump into each other, he accidentally touches her crotch with his hand and she knees him in the crotch.

Up in triptych openings on the wall, Jalet and Neyskens represent Adam and Eve as they stand semi-naked, evoking the iconography of medieval paintings. Svensson and Vladyslav kiss, and the rest of the stage action freezes, as if someone had pressed the pause button. Dudley, meanwhile, lists things that make her happy into the PA system: 'the morning light, sleeping in, smelling the back of a baby's neck, the smell of fresh washing, cucumber sandwiches, riding a bike with no hands, coming home, my mother, my father, my husband, my child...' Dudley then begins to sing the opening of 'Somewhere over the rainbow' from the film *The Wizard of Oz* (1939).

Svensson addresses the audience, giving the 'worldwide weather forecast' and introduces herself as Deborah Rainbow. The bad weather seems confined to areas of recent military conflict, civil war and violence: Belfast, the Balkan, Chechnya, Afghanistan, Israel, Iraq and Iran. A row of angels advance, hands clasped behind their backs and heads bowing down, and they get pummelled and knocked down by an oblivious Svensson as she points to an imaginary world map. Dudley releases something like sleeping gas, which causes the protagonists and angels to fall asleep. As Leboutte starts to sing 'Ave Maria', the dancers rise and face the audience with their hands clasped behind their backs. They harmonise with Leboutte, but the chords are somewhat dissonant and unusual. Dudley puts on a raincoat and protective ear-defenders, and repeatedly smashes a hammer loudly and at a fast, but steady pace, onto a block of metal, thus creating a pulse. The pulse ignores the pulse and rhythm of the coinciding *a capella* song. The dancers commence a *staccato* movement phrase, executing one movement on every pulse. They repeatedly descend to the floor and get back up. The tempo of the pulse seems to be too fast for the dancers and their movements become jerky, as if their bodies are manipulated and abused by an external force. When Dudley starts speeding up the pulse, the dancers give the impression of being exhausted, and one by one they fall onto the floor with a loud and desperate scream, accompanied by the sound of breaking glass. When the last dancer has died, Dudley puts down the hammer and takes off the headphones. Afterwards, Woods wakes up and looks around at the scattered bodies in horror. He grabs the hammer from Dudley, condemning her actions with a 'Thou shalt not kill'.

By focusing on matters central to humanity—life, death, love, war, hope, desperation—Cherkaoui brings the issue of religion down to the very question of belief and human experience itself away from any particular religious perspectives or doctrines. The work can thus be seen as Cherkaoui's initial exploration of a transreligious perspective, beginning with the music and iconography of the Christian tradition as a focal point. While these elements may seem familiar to Western audiences when they encounter them, Cherkaoui is asking spectators to look again and invites them into a macro-dramaturgical engagement with their own sense of identity and community.

MUSIC IN *FOI*

Cherkaoui stated that music was to a large extent the starting point in the development of *Foi* (Cherkaoui qtd. in Capilla Flamenca 8); therefore, it is necessary to learn more about the musical elements that are joined together in the work. For the creation of *Foi*, an interesting collaboration took place with artists specialised in an area that Cherkaoui was fascinated by and wanted to learn about. Having sung 'Stabat Mater' with Damien Jalet in *Rien de Rien*, Cherkaoui began a search for new, additional partners to shed a different light on ancient, orally transmitted music, which would become a key dramaturgical focus in his work throughout the rest of the decade, notably in *Myth* through collaboration with Ensemble Micrologus and *Apocrifu* with the Corsican group A Filetta. In *Foi*, the fourteenth-century music of the Ars Nova, performed by Capilla Flamenca, is juxtaposed to orally transmitted music sung by the other performers. In preparation for the creation of *Foi*, Cherkaoui studied and researched medieval music with Snellings and Capilla Flamenca for one year. Ars Nova music originated in France, spread throughout Europe, and was further developed in Italy. Rediscovered written sources have caught the interest of contemporary musicians and musicologists, and Capilla Flamenca performs music based on these sources. In an interview in 2004, Snellings explained that the main characteristic of this music is the autonomy of each musical line, resulting in polyphonic compositions in which a rhythmical complexity is created through a refined treatment of each part's temporal subdivisions. The *Trecento* composers in Italy emphasised virtuosity and new harmonies, leading to a highly refined tonal language. This musical innovation left its mark in Ghent, one of the large urban centres of Flanders, where a vast number of local Ars Nova scores have been found. These scores include motets, mass movements, courtly songs, such as the *ballade*, *virelai*, and *rondeau*, and courtly dances. During the performance of *Foi*, various types of Ars Nova music are performed by a quartet of male singers and three musicians of Capilla Flamenca, playing the lute, fiddle, recorder, bagpipe, and percussion (Snellings qtd. in Capilla Flamenca 12; Snellings).

Music that is orally transmitted is the second source of music in *Foi*, and can be considered a continuation of Cherkaoui's work from *Rien de Rien* and *d'avant* (2002). Leboutte performs three songs from the rich repertoire of traditional music for Holy Week in Italy. This music continues to be played today in the villages of southern Italy, sung by non-professional singers in Easter processions. She clarified in interview that the aesthetic characteristics of this typical rural singing are found in the performance method. The voice is used in a rather forced way and sounds loud and clear, without the use of the head voice. More than the melody or the text, it is the type of sound, the timbre and the colour that the young people of the village learn from the older singers. For instance, in the songs of Sardinian shepherds, the voices imitate animal sounds, for example, from goats or sheep. The songs are also performed in a very flexible rhythm. *Melismata* are added at the whim of the performer, as well as a long coda and *rinforzando* towards the end of a song (Leboutte qtd. in Capilla Flamenca 5; Leboutte).

The music of *Foi* was recorded and made commercially available on CD in 2003, followed later as a model by the music CD release of *Myth* in 2007. The booklet accompanying the CD includes texts by Cherkaoui and the musical collaborators, as well as the lyrics to the songs, translated in Dutch, French and English, juxtaposed to photographic images from the respective scenes from the performance. The availability of these song texts has been important in that it allowed me as a spectator to relive aspects of the performance to a certain extent, focusing on the meaning of the songs, which often added an unexpected dramaturgical layer. Crucially, in the booklet, Cherkaoui indicates that *Foi* makes a macro-dramaturgical link between historical events from the Middle Ages, such as the crusades, and recent developments like the war in Iraq.

> The question arises of whether so very much has changed since the Middle Ages. We look back condescendingly at their 'barbarism', while sometimes refusing to open our eyes to the analogous brutalities of the present day. (Cherkaoui qtd. in Capilla Flamenca 8)

Having briefly considered Cherkaoui's artistic concerns and methods when creating *Foi*, it can be surmised that the work thrives on the juxtaposition of diverging musicalities. The abundance and polyphony of different voices in *Foi* is visualised in a simultaneous juxtaposition of choreographic images and religious iconography and will come to stand for the work's multiplicity of influences in creation, combining stories, songs, choreographed movements and theatrical images. Detailed description of *Foi* provides evidence of its multi-layered construction, incorporating narrative, song, choreographed movement, gesture and visual pictography.

In the scene where Leboutte holds up the photo of Jalet as if he is looking for her son, she sings the *a capella* traditional song, 'Passione de Guilianello'. It is the passion story of Christ's suffering, from the viewpoint of Mary, his mother. 'Dimmi se'l mio figlio è vivo or morto', she sings, which can be translated as 'Tell me if my son is alive or dead' (Capilla Flamenca 16). Her voice is deep, piercing and urgent. Jalet, as angel, visualises the sounds coming out of her mouth with his hands, and harmonises with Leboutte. Neyskens sings the third voice, as one of a group of dancers who balance arching back in a bridge stance on hands and feet, their heads hanging upside down facing the audience. Their elbows collapse and they restore the bridge position repeatedly, effectuating a continuing sense of movement in this otherwise static position. The sound flows freely out of Neyskens's open mouth, while she maintains this awkward and challenging movement, indicating sufficient relaxation of the vocal chords and complete control of the breath. This choreographic image serves to tune the spectator into the voices on an affective level, with the aim of opening up macro-dramaturgical connections between images regularly circulated in the broadcast media of suffering mothers who have lost their sons in war zones, for example, in the Middle East, and Mary's suffering at the loss of her son in the Bible. However, it needed the religious community of women in the southern Italian town of Giulianello to vocalise the female perspective in this Bible story. By setting this Christian sung lament within the scene of the aftermath of a disaster or war, Cherkaoui then macro-dramaturgically opens up the transreligious connections to the singing of laments in other religious traditions.

Ómarsdóttir then dons an oversized black leather jacket and a woolly hat, which is pulled halfway over her face, covering her eyes. She weakly mutters repeatedly: 'I'm sorry. I'm really, really sorry. I promise I'll be a good boy'. Jalet towers over her and slowly pulls the hat off, while Ómarsdóttir screams in a raw, piercing voice. She sings the opening lines of the Icelandic lullaby 'Sofðu unga ástin mín', while Jalet and Kim manhandle her, throw her to the ground and twist her into painful looking positions. This is then juxtaposed with the soft early English lullaby 'Lulay, lulay', which depicts an unusual view of the nativity scene: Mary rocks her baby to sleep and reminisces of the words spoken to her by the archangel Gabriel. At the end of the scene, Ómarsdóttir falls off the stage into the orchestra pit. Wagemans lifts her out and cares for her, carefully removing the leather jacket from her.

Leboutte starts singing 'Li Lamenti', 'a real cry out with Arab characteristics from the village of Grotte, Sicily', pointing at the transcultural influences on the musical development in the Mediterranean region (Leboutte qtd. in Capilla Flamenca 2). The other dancers sing the responses as a choir, facing the wall, while Jalet extends his movements into the singing of the second solo part of 'Li Lamenti'. His voice is raw and piercing. Ómarsdóttir relentlessly scribbles the lyrics of the song she is about to sing in chalk on the back wall. Wagemans walks with Jalet, holding his hand, and offers him his jacket. Jalet, with his eyes closed, recites a story in French about the experiences of a survivor of the nuclear attack on Hiroshima. He holds a Braille book and moves his fingers over the text, suggesting that the attack has left him blind. Svensson is wearing boxing gloves with the American stars and stripes printed on them, and she has her eyes taped shut. She punches Vladyslav, who is suspended upside down on the wall, in the stomach (Fig. 4.1).

Ómarsdóttir begins to sing the Icelandic lullaby 'Sofðu unga ástin mín'. While she is balancing with her pelvis or limbs on the Jalet's feet, he rocks her as if he were a baby's cradle and moves across the floor on his back. In these awkward positions, at a certain point even hanging upside down between his legs, she performs baby-like movements with her arms and legs, indirect and in free-flow, gathering towards the centre of her body. The movements influence her breathing; it becomes heavy, which in turn has an effect on her singing voice. The raw, scraping sound of the voice provides a new context for interpretation of the movements. Ómarsdóttir introduced this Icelandic lullaby to Cherkaoui as part of the creative process. However, usually only the first verse of the lullaby, in which a mother comforts her child and lulls it to sleep, is sung by

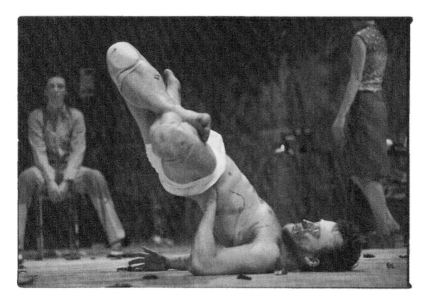

Fig. 4.1   Damien Jalet in *Foi* (Photo by Kurt Van Der Elst/kvde.be)

mothers to their infants: 'Sleep my young love, outside the rain is crying. Mama will watch over your gold, an old leg and a stone case. We should not stay awake in dark nights' (Capilla Flamenca 31). Ómarsdóttir discovered that there are three verses in total, and that the lullaby originates in ancient Icelandic Sagas. The text of the second and third verse is much darker and more desperate, referring to death, darkness, love, loss, tears and absence: 'Darkness knows many things, my mind is empty. Often I have looked into the black sand. Dead, deep cracks sound in the glacier. Sleep long and peacefully, it is best to wake up late Mæðum, I will teach you now, as the day quickly passes, about human love, loss, tears and absence' (Capilla Flamenca 31). The legend behind this lullaby is that it was sung by a female slave who wanted to protect her child from slavery by ending its life. Ómarsdóttir found it a fascinating phenomenon that many Icelandic mothers sing a lullaby to their babies, which in its second and third verses refers to a mother killing her child (Ómarsdóttir). She succeeds in transferring the dark atmosphere from the content of the lullaby to her singing and dancing.

Foi is a work in which movement, speech, song and instrumental music are highly integrated and no hierarchy is distinguishable between the art forms of dance, theatre and music. In this work, Cherkaoui tackles big cultural questions: religion, language, history and national identity—themes that he would continue to research in other works during this first decade of the new millennium. While and after I watched *Foi*, I reflected on my experience as a spectator. I realised that I had no means of accounting for the strong affective, physical responses I felt to the powerful sections of the performance. I had goose bumps, I cried, I cringed, I smiled, I laughed out loud, I moved with the dancers, I felt heavy and weighed down, I felt lifted and weightless. Cherkaoui provides a dramaturgical rationale for this:

> Besides beautiful, funny or more calm moments, there are more aggressive scenes in Foi, which could make the audience feel somewhat uncomfortable. The idea is to sketch a complete picture of human behaviour. Within all these moments of harmony and violence, survival is the most important theme. The urge is crucial for the true meaning hidden in the word conviction – even more than belief or spirituality. (Cherkaoui qtd. in Capilla Flamenca 8)

The etymological root of the word 'conviction' that Cherkaoui refers to is the Latin 'vincere' or 'to conquer', connecting the basis of religion to conquest. In all of *Foi's* complexity and persuasive polyvocality, I was deeply implicated in the performance as a spectator and felt addressed directly and interpellated.

By reducing the issue of religion to the question of 'What do you believe in?' Cherkaoui focuses the attention on human experience. In a stark post-trauma environment, evocative of 9/11, *Foi* shows its protagonists searching for moral and spiritual guidance using varying strategies and levels of success. For example, Woods resorts to sanctimony and bible bashing, while Dudley, struck by grief, turns violent towards others. Both through the emphasis on stories, the human stories underpinning familiar Christian iconography, and through the affective responses he solicits, Cherkaoui is asking spectators to look and think again. Cherkaoui's transreligious macro dramaturgy begins in this work with Christianity itself: by offering late-medieval musical perspectives, as well as those from the oral tradition in the Mediterranean region, he invites spectators to engage anew with ideas that have fundamentally shaped Western ways of thinking. These are gently juxtaposed with secular elements, such as lullabies and love songs, and those pertaining to other cultures, such as Korean and Chinese songs. His approach to Christianity is decentred, occupying both insider and outsider perspective. Where *Foi* was created in the wake of the 9/11 terrorist attacks and takes the aftermath of a disaster as its starting point, in his later work *Apocrifu*, Cherkaoui provides a direct challenge to the religious fundamentalisms at the heart of these attacks.

CONTEXTUALISING AND THEORISING FUNDAMENTALISMS

One of the key events to provide a contextual backdrop to Cherkaoui's choreographic explorations of religious themes is the Salman Rushdie affair. Controversy arose over the British Indian writer's 1988 novel *The Satanic Verses*, in the form of hostility and violent reactions by some Muslim groups. In 1989, the Ayatollah Khomeini of Iran issued a *fatwa* or death sentence against Rushdie. The issue at the heart of the dispute was the tension between, on the one hand, freedom of speech as the epitome of Western libertarian values and, on the other hand, Muslim concerns about the dishonouring of the prophet Mohammed. The title of the book refers to verses that were allegedly dictated to the prophet by the devil and were later removed from the Qur'an, and is regarded by some Muslims to be blasphemous. A number of people involved in the publication and distribution of the novel were killed, and several attempts were made on Rushdie's life, causing him to live in exile for a considerable time. Literary scholar Margaret Scanlan regrets that the Rushdie affair has largely overshadowed the author's work itself, and has prevented conventional literary criticism of *The Satanic Verses*, stating that 'history has violated the boundaries of this fiction' (231). She evaluates the central premise of the book, which is 'to imagine the possibility, which lurks in an apocryphal tradition, that the Qu'ran might be an edited text, that Muhammed might briefly have allowed into it a few verses of satanic origin', as being 'harmless enough' to postmodern readers who are used to stories being retold in new registers (Scanlan 230). It is in this respect that Rushdie's novel bears relevance to the study of Cherkaoui's work. It will be argued in the latter half of this chapter that his work *Apocrifu* choreographically represents Holy texts as man-made, fluid and subject to revision and editing, thereby undermining religious fundamentalisms that consider Holy texts to literally be 'the Word of God'.

There is an interesting branch of literary scholarship that usefully attempts to articulate Rushdie's stance towards fundamentalism. Analysing Rushdie's novel *The Moor's Last Sigh*, literary scholar Dohra Ahmad interrogates the term fundamentalism within the context of modernity, globalisation and late capitalism. She proposes the pluralisation of the term—fundamentalisms—to indicate Rushdie's stance 'that fundamentalist mindsets infect not only Islam but also Hinduism, Christianity, Marxism, modern art, and for that matter even the doctrine of hybridity that so many of us would prefer to view as redemptively flexible' (Ahmad 2). Perhaps the relative absence of Islam and Muslim characters in this later novel occurred in response to the 1989 *fatwa* following *The Satanic Verses*, in the sense that afterwards Rushdie dissociated himself directly from the Islamic world. However, the implicit meaning is that 'Islam is only one of many rigid, totalizing visions that claim to rely on an eternal truth' (Ahmad 2). In his choreographic representations of religious themes, Cherkaoui highlights a range of fundamentalisms across Christianity, Judaism and Islam, and thus echoes Rushdie's indiscriminate critique of religious fundamentalisms.

In September 2005 and the ensuing months, another controversy dominated the news in the Western world, repeating similar arguments to those that fuelled the Rushdie affair. The Danish newspaper *Jyllands-Posten* published cartoons depicting Mohammed—an act which is considered blasphemous in Islam, even without considering that in one of the cartoons the prophet was depicted as a suicide bomber. The cartoons aimed to stimulate the debate about the critical evaluation of Islam as part of free speech. The act was condemned by Islamic groups in Denmark and around the world as insensitive, Islamophobic and sacrilegious. Violent protests by these groups followed. It is thought that *Jyllands-Posten*'s campaign was a response to the assassination of Dutch film maker Theo Van Gogh by a Dutch Muslim of Moroccan origin in 2004, following Van Gogh's collaboration with Ayaan Hirsi Ali, a Somali-born writer living and working in the Netherlands as a politician. Van Gogh and Hirsi Ali produced the film *Submission* in 2004, which highlighted and criticised the abuse of women in Islamic societies. The film features scenes in which verses from the Qur'an proclaiming men's superiority over women were painted on a woman's naked skin. Poignantly, Cherkaoui's work *Apocrifu* also features a scene in which one dancer paints onto another dancer's naked torso—albeit Japanese calligraphy rather than Qur'anic verses.

In March 2006, a group of writers, including Rushdie and Hirsi Ali, signed a political manifesto published in the French magazine *Charlie Hebdo*, entitled 'Together Facing the New Totalitarianism':

> After having overcome fascism, Nazism, and Stalinism, the world now faces a new global totalitarian threat: Islamism. We, writers, journalists, intellectuals, call for resistance to religious totalitarianism and for the promotion of freedom, equal opportunity and secular values for all. (BBC News *Writers' Statement on Cartoons*)

These values are deemed by the signatories of the manifesto to be 'universal'. 'Islamism', they claim,

> [...] is nurtured by fear and frustration. Preachers of hatred play on these feelings to build the forces with which they can impose a world where liberty is crushed and inequality reigns. [...] We reject the "cultural relativism" which implies an acceptance that men and women of Muslim culture are deprived of the right to equality, freedom and secularism in the name of the respect for certain cultures and traditions. (BBC News *Writers' Statement on Cartoons*)

However, anthropologist David Perusek assesses the signatories' dismissal of cultural relativism in the context of the 'free-floating signifier' he argues it has become in postmodern argumentation (830). Their rejection of the concept, Perusek argues, is not the result of their being 'narrow minded absolutist (they are not)', but of a careful evaluation of contemporary anthropology's misuse of the term (831). He astutely notes

> that those signatories and all who share their view have themselves long cultivated and relied upon the intellectual stance of cultural relativism in order to interpret and, in many cases, re-present the world around them [...] [and] that they themselves would be intellectually paralyzed without it. (Perusek 831)

Andrew Shryock, in his introduction to the edited volume *Islamophobia/ Islamophilia*, heavily criticises the manifesto as being 'simplistic and alarmist' (5) and problematises its conflating of Islam and Islamism, a supposed ideology which is, however, scantily defined. In the manifesto, the authors defensively, and—in Shryock's eyes—ineffectively, renounce the label 'islamophobic':

> We refuse to renounce our critical spirit out of fear of being accused of "Islamophobia", a wretched concept that confuses criticism of Islam as a religion and stigmatisation of those who believe in it. (BBC News *Writers' Statement on Cartoons*)

Overall, Shryock argues for a less essentialised understanding of Islam, given that it is hard to draw clear lines between Self and Other in an increasingly globalised world.

Complex debates are held about these developments, invoking concepts and phrases such as fundamentalism, freedom of speech, blasphemy, new totalitarianism and Islamophobia. These redefinitions and, sometimes, misuses of the terminology indicate that the debates themselves are increasingly complex, with arguments and counterarguments continuously being thrown backwards and forwards. There is no straightforward right or wrong. It is in this context that Cherkaoui's choreographic negotiations of religion should be evaluated as those of someone whose life has been located at the crossroads of religious tensions in Western Europe, particularly in relation to the rise of the populist radical right in Flanders. The rest of this chapter will argue that Cherkaoui positions himself very carefully in this myriad of voices through subtle choreographic strategies in *Apocrifu*.

CHOREOGRAPHING THE INTERTEXTUALITY OF RELIGIOUS TEXTS IN *APOCRIFU*

This section will present a detailed reading of a brief excerpt of *Apocrifu* as a critique of religious discourse. Without discussing the work in its entirety, quick access to its dramaturgical content can be gained through analysis of the use of props and the work's title. Throughout the work a large number of leather-bound books are moved and manipulated in a variety of metaphorical acts. The sudden sound of a book being dropped on the floor interrupts a virtuosic solo by Dimitri Jourde, who undulates with sequential and circular motions down to and up from the floor to the *a capella* rendition of a traditional Mediterranean 'Kyrie Eleison', performed live on stage by the male vocal ensemble A Filetta. Cherkaoui holds a stack of books and drops them one by one, using the books as stepping stones to create a path. However, the books as stepping stones seem to only allow him to go to a certain point and no further. Later, he dances a solo where he elevates an open book above his head in awe. Classical arabesques and pirouettes are juxtaposed to rolling on the floor and contortionist kneeling yoga poses, all the while the hand holding the book remaining the highest point, the axis around which his whole body pivots. Cherkaoui looks up to the book with an inquisitive gaze and moves his right hand up to the left, pulling the book down and pushing it all the way to the floor. As soon as the right hand lets go, the book rises up to the highest point again, pulling Cherkaoui's body along into an upright standing position. The book hovers in front of his face, as if he is reading it, and—still engrossed in the book's content, eyes fixed—it directs Cherkaoui through the space, causing him to arch back all the way down to the floor, around and up, travelling across the stage, oblivious to his surroundings. Then, the book comes down crushing his face, so that he cannot see where he is going. Finally, Cherkaoui's solo ends with the book leading him into a whirling pattern resembling a Sufi dervish dance. At the end of the performance, Cherkaoui, and fellow performers Jourde and Yasuyuki Shuto each pierce a book with a sword, suggesting an act of renunciation of the written word.

The title of the work refers to the Apocrypha, which can be defined as those Christian writings that were excluded from the canons of the Old and New Testament. The distinction between the Apocryphal as opposed to the Canonical gospels is believed to have led to the word 'apocryphal' taking on meanings such as unauthentic, spurious, fictitious, invented, imagined (rather than true or genuine), or implying a mysterious or dubious source of origin. These negative, derogatory connotations denote an attitude which fails to take into account the values of the texts themselves and the subjective and arbitrary processes involved in the creation of the distinction between Apocrypha and Canon. This seems, to theological scholar Helmut Koester, largely misplaced. The title *Apocrifu* sets the scene for Cherkaoui's dramaturgical concerns in this work, namely the processes and stakes involved in writing the canonical religious texts and the implications of their elevation for the religion's followers, which, it is implicitly suggested, may lead to religious fundamentalism. In a broader sense, this theme resonates with Cherkaoui's historiographical distrust of the written word and his transcultural renunciation of the idea of cultures as discrete, pure and impenetrable. He explains: 'Once they are printed, words can't evolve anymore. I find this definitive side of ink and paper intimidating. Every truth is related to a certain time. It is possible that the truth of what is written today becomes a lie of my future thoughts' (qtd. in Cools 91).

Cherkaoui, Jourde and Shuto face each other and pass three leather-bound books between each other: the Bible, the Torah and the Qur'an, the Holy books of three historically linked world religions. Cherkaoui randomly opens up his book; Jourde and Shuto follow suit and hold their open books next to his in order to compare them. They move so that they are standing behind one another with their books held high one behind the other, so that it looks like a unified image of a single man holding up a single book. As the men go through the same motions of lowering the book and folding it across their chests, there are some slight delays and accelerations, so that the image multiplies, evoking the iconography of Shiva. Non-matching pairs of hands grab hold of the books and open them. Torsos lean from side to side allowing for the men to scrutinise, flick through and skim read all three books. The loops of non-matching arms weave in and out of each other, like a magician's trick, so that no one knows which book belonged to whom anymore. This theatrical image, with the bearded Shuto standing in front of the other two dancers, his dark eyes gazing solemnly into the audience, evokes medieval Orthodox icons of Christ Pantocrator, or Christ the Almighty, usually depicted clutching the Gospels in his left arm and using the right hand to perform a blessing. The image represents Christ as the all-knowing and fair judge of humanity. In Cherkaoui's new choreographic iconography, the shapeshifting and multiplication of the Christ figure into a holy trinity of its own, suggests that there are similarities between the three holy texts of these interrelated religions and that their associated holy figures recur across each of them. This is confirmed by what happens next (Fig. 4.2).

Cherkaoui recites a speech by Reverend Jay Smith, a researcher of the sources of the scriptures of the Bible and the Qur'an, which was taken from a video clip on YouTube, bluntly entitled 'Is the Qur'an corrupted? Biblical characters in the Qur'an', and then memorised and choreographed. The speech highlights the intertextual connections between

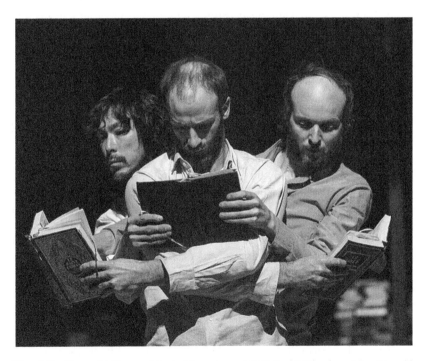

Fig. 4.2 Yasuyuki Shuto, Dimitri Jourde and Sidi Larbi Cherkaoui in *Apocrifu* (Photo by Foteini Christofilopoulou/www.foteini.com)

the two Holy texts and editorial amendments made when the texts were reproduced throughout the centuries. Smith's aim is to undermine fundamentalist readings of the Qur'an as 'the word of God'. Instead, he argues that the text has its origins in Jewish Talmudic and Christian Apocryphal writings. Cherkaoui, too, seems deeply suspicious of religious fundamentalism, and choreographs the intertextuality of the Bible, the Torah and the Qur'an in the trio for three male dancers described above.

'It's been fascinating when I read the Qur'an, because when I read the Qur'an I find a lot of the characters in the Qur'an are the same characters I find in my Bible. You have Abraham-Abrahim; you have Moses-Moyse; you have David-Dauda, Jesus-Isa, John the Baptist-Yahya [Shuto flicks through a few pages of an open book, while Cherkaoui alternately points at this book and another]. But it's fascinating when you look at the stories in the Qur'an; they do not parallel the stories I have in my Bible. I always scratch my head [Shuto scratches Cherkaoui's head] and say, hold on a minute, where do these stories come from? They don't parallel the same material [Cherkoui wags both index fingers from side to side to signal "no"]. Let's give some examples; let's go back to Cain and Abel. Cain and Abel, in Sura 5 Aya 31, Cain has just killed his brother Abel [Jourde mimics stabbing Shuto]; he doesn't know what to do with the body. He looks over and he sees a raven scratching the ground and he says, well I'm going to follow what the raven does and he buries his brother like he sees the raven doing. Terrific story, but it's not in my Bible [Jourde frantically flicks through one of the books and then throws his arms up in exasperation]. So, where does it come from? We know exactly where it comes from, we've done source criticism on these accounts and we can go back to them and we find that in the Targum of Jonathan-ben-Uzziah, also the Targum of Jerusalem and also the Pirke-Rabbi Eleazar [Jourde and Shuto forcibly thrust three books onto Cherkaoui's upward-facing palm one by one, causing him to collapse slightly under the weight of each book], three different accounts from the second century which talk about the same story, it seems that these were borrowed from those accounts. What's interesting is the next verse, because in verse 32 it suddenly changes. There's a reference there about the blood of Abel and then it mentions that [Jourde and Shuto join in in unison, their heads suddenly appearing on each of Cherkaoui's shoulders] "He who takes the blood of one, takes the bloods of all, and he who saves the blood of one, saves the bloods

of all" This is a very popular reference used by Muslims today to stipulate that Islam is a religion of peace, because they don't take people's
blood [Shuto mimics strangling Jourde by grabbing his throat with both
hands]; they actually save people by not taking their blood [Jourde and
Shuto hug each other]. The difficulty is, what is it doing after verse 31?
It seems to almost be a redemptive account; it doesn't belong in that
story. Until you realise that in the fourth [Shuto interrupts and says
'fifth' into Cherkaoui's ear], the fifth century, excuse me, there was a
scribe who was re-writing the Targum of Jonathan-ben-Uzziah, and as
he was re-writing it, as scribes do, in the margins he actually puts an editorial comment on the blood of Abel, and he mentions that [Jourde and
Shuto join in in unison] "he who takes the blood of one, takes the blood
of all, and he who saves the blood of one, saves the blood of all". Now,
when that was incorporated into the Bar Sanhedrin Chapter 4 Verse 5 in
the fifth century, that story of Cain and Abel and the raven was then followed by this editorial comment on the blood of Abel, taken from that
editorial comment in the margins, incorporated into the Bar Sanhedrin
Chapter 4 Verse 5. And then both that story plus the editorial comment
were then incorporated into the Qur'an in Sura 5 Aya 31 and 32. Now
what does that tell you? [Cherkaoui pauses and suspiciously moves his
eyes from side to side, while Jourde holds his book in front of his nose
and mouth so that only his eyes are visible, which he, too, moves from
side to side] I know what it tells me. It tells me that we now know where
these stories come from. They do not come from God; were not divinely
inspired; they were basically written by men'.

In the YouTube clip, Smith talks at an extraordinarily quick pace, and
this is mimicked by Cherkaoui, who sometimes struggles and needs to
pause to breathe or swallow. During the recounting of the text Jourde
and Shuto make comical interventions into the text. When Cherkaoui
says 'I always scratch my head', Shuto scratches Cherkaoui's head. When
Cherkaoui mentions the story of Cain and Abel, Jourde mimics stabbing
Shuto. The three men recite the phrase 'He who takes the blood of one,
takes the bloods of all, and he who saves the blood of one, saves the
bloods of all' in unison, gazing at the audience in bewilderment. When
Smith in the YouTube video makes a mistake and mixes up the centuries,
this is translated in the choreography as Shuto interrupting Cherkaoui
and correcting him. When Smith in his speech uses the rhetoric device of
posing the question 'Now what does that tell you?' followed by a pregnant pause, Cherkaoui pauses and suspiciously moves his eyes from side

to side, while Jourde holds his book in front of his nose and mouth so that only his eyes are visible, which he, too, moves from side to side.

The key point Smith makes in this text is that these religious texts are in fact man-made and subject to error in copying, and indeed to editorial revisions. Smith published the same research in a more scholarly written online article entitled 'Is the Qur'an the Word of God?' on the debate. org website, which is owned by the Hyde Park Christian Fellowship, 'an informal network of Christian researchers in the UK, whose primary interest is the academic study of all issues relevant to Islam and Christianity'. It is problematic, although perhaps not deliberate, that the majority of texts published on the website are by Western, non-Muslim writers, with a great many by Smith alone, rendering it primarily a representation of Islam through Western eyes. An underlying ethnocentric agenda of critiquing the way in which some Muslims read their Holy text as the Word of God can also be felt. While for a Christian this may be an understandable entry into civilised debate with Islam, it superimposes a Western, post-Enlightenment, moderate approach to religious texts and therefore fails to understand the role of the Qur'an from within Islam. This is in line with Arjun Appadurai's term 'ideoscapes', which indicates that the ideology and world view of the Enlightenment have undergone a worldwide diaspora, but have become detached from the internal logic of its original context. Hence, this Western ideology has been appropriated incompletely and become lost in translation. Therefore, Appadurai seems to allude to the limitations of a continued use of this set of ideas as 'correct'.

Nevertheless, Cherkaoui may have selected to cite this text in *Apocrifu* precisely because it undermines the power and supremacy of the written religious word. Smith contends that his critical analysis of the evidence of man-made interventions in the text of the Qur'an seems to 'point away from a divine authorship and point towards a more plausible explanation; that the Qur'an is simply a collection of disparate sources borrowed from surrounding pieces of literature, folk tales, and oral traditions' (Smith). This seems to be a message that Cherkaoui can subscribe to, although at the same time he implicitly keeps his distance from Smith's other possible agendas and ethnocentric bias by using, not his own, but Smith's words; by mimicking Smith's pace of speech, which adds to a strangely comical effect in his reciting of the text; and by choreographing the other two performers' comical interventions.

Thatamanil recognises that the notion of the transreligious interrogates the legitimacy of the expression of divine disclosure in the scriptures of a certain religious tradition. 'Isn't the theologian bound and constrained by what his or her tradition believes to be God's full and final self-disclosure?' (Thatamanil 359). He rebuts the potential criticism inherent in this line of inquiry by pointing at the transreligious nature of religions through history; the early Christians had to simultaneously build on and distance themselves from existing insights from the established, surrounding religious traditions and were therefore constructively comparative all along. Overall, transreligious theology does not accept a certain set of scriptures as the full and final set of answers to life's questions. Cherkaoui, in his creative exploration of religious themes, likewise seeks to test the limits of the validity of particular religious texts and the notion of religions being in a continuous process of transformation through encounters with the Other. He actively seeks out these kinds of transcultural, transreligious encounters for himself at the basis of each work.

The availability of Smith's speech on YouTube needs to be evaluated critically. On the one hand, in line with the optimistic promise held by the semiotic democracy, it could be considered beneficial to encourage debate between Christians and Muslims using such a popular medium. On the other hand, because YouTube is a medium which is relatively unedited and users are able to comment relatively freely, any such debates occur in a vacuum; are rarely constructive; and border on hate speech. A survey of the user comments since the clip was posted in November 2006 indicates that Smith's video evoked many heated responses by YouTube users representing different religions and ideologies. The relative anonymity of the users allows for fairly injurious language. Sometimes the hate speech is directed at Smith, sometimes at other users, and sometimes at no one in particular. Often the comments bear no relation to Smith's argument and slip into a religious fundamentalism which is precisely what he may have been arguing against. This illustrates that the premise of Western, post-Enlightenment scholarship is no longer viable in an increasingly globalised world, or a 'modernity at large' in the Appaduraian sense, where people have free and unmediated access to information, opinions and debate and in principle everyone has the right and means to voice their opinion.

In the YouTube context, where notions of subject and object are problematised, and website officials merely use an automatised system to identify offensive language, there is scope for hate speech to be uttered relatively uncensored. In Judith Butler's *Excitable Speech*, which discusses 'linguistic vulnerability' and 'injurious speech', her overall argument is that it is impossible to regulate hate speech through censorship, precisely because this assumes a universal notion of what is acceptable (*Excitable Speech* 30–43). Instead, she argues that language is politically and socially useful, precisely to the extent that it is excitable, or out of control, in play, performative, act-like (Butler *Excitable Speech*). Butler's writing practice tends to resignify language, by presenting it in a new light. Similarly, Cherkaoui's appropriation of Smith's discourse can be seen as a resignification, in the sense that Cherkaoui 'playfully' keeps his distance from Smith's apparent ethnocentric agenda and association with online hate speech, which ensues from this kind of unmonitored digital religious discourse. This resignification of Smith's speech opens up renewed possibility for reflection and debate, but on Cherkaoui's own terms and in his own artistic language. He selects a piece of the text which he as a postcolonial figure can subscribe to and which works in the overall dramaturgy of *Apocrifu*, i.e. Smith's critique of the elevation of canonical religious texts by these religions' followers. However, Cherkaoui subjects the YouTube speech to postmodern distancing strategies, and thereby distances himself from Smith's ethnocentric bias and the ensuing online hate speech. Overall, Cherkaoui's choreography suggests that fundamentalist, literal interpretations of religious texts can be violent, and, via the internet, also potentially volatile.

The aim of this chapter was to evaluate the ways in which Cherkaoui intervenes in the debates on religious fundamentalism and Islamophobia through his choreographic negotiations of religious themes. *Apocrifu* choreographically represents the intertextuality of the Bible, Qur'an and Torah drawing attention to the man-made nature of religious texts, thereby undermining religious fundamentalisms and the proclaimed power of the written religious Word. Cherkaoui negotiates his authorial voice as a choreographer by working selectively with Smith's ethnocentric speech and subjecting it to distancing strategies, including humour. In line with Butler's (*Excitable Speech*) warning not to carry out censorship against injurious speech and Appadurai's questioning of seemingly universalised Western values, Cherkaoui resignifies this excitable speech 'at large' in the digital age in a playful way. He therefore demonstrates that he is carefully balancing the diverging arguments that infuse the debates on religious fundamentalism, conveying an extremely subtle and considerate stance that does not put blame on any one religious group. Recent reflections on transreligious theology have begun to envisage the notion of the post religious, with theology's home moving from religious institutions to the academy:

> Suppose for a moment that transreligious theology eventually takes its (rightful, I think) place in the secular academy [...] Is it not then the case that transreligious theology is welcomed and sustained within the secular academy with such wholeheartedness that its parasitic relationship with positive religious traditions falls away? I think so. In that situation, we arrive at postreligious theology, or nonreligious theology—that is, theology that makes intellectual sense with no specific religious tradition at its root and remains socially viable with no living religious institution for support. (Wildman 247)

Through his transreligious dramaturgy, Cherkaoui uses the performing arts as an equally viable site of transreligious exploration and reflection, inviting spectators to participate in this never-ending hermeneutic endeavour through their ongoing engagement with his works' micro and macro dramaturgies.

BIBLIOGRAPHY

Ahmad, Dohra. '"This Fundo Stuff Is Really Something New": Fundamentalism and Hybridity in The Moor's Last Sigh'. *The Yale Journal of Criticism*. 18.1. (2005): 1–20. Print.

Appadurai, Arjun. *Modernity at Large: Cultural Dimensions of Globalization*. Minneapolis: University of Minnesota Press, 1996. Print.

BBC News. 'Full Text: Writers' Statement on Cartoons'. 2006. Web. Accessed: 6 July 2012. <http://news.bbc.co.uk/1/hi/world/europe/4764730.stm>.

Butler, Judith. *Excitable Speech: A Politics of the Performative*. London: Routledge, 1997. Print.

Capilla Flamenca – Les Ballets C. de la B. *Foi: Ars Nova, Oral Traditional Music & More*. Leuven: Capilla Flamenca, 2003. Booklet with CD.

Cools, Guy. *In-Between Dance Cultures: On the Migratory Artistic Identity of Sidi Larbi Cherkaoui and Akram Khan*. Antennae Series. Amsterdam: Valiz, 2015. Print.

Faber, Roland. 'Der Transreligiöse Diskurs. Zu Einer Theologie Transformativer Prozesse'. *Polylog*. 9. (2002): 65–94. Print.

Koester, Helmut. 'Apocryphal and Canonical Gospels'. *The Harvard Theological Review*. 73.1/2. (1980): 105–130. Print.

Micrologus. *Myth—Sidi Larbi Cherkaoui: The Music*. 2007. Booklet with CD.

Perusek, David. 'Grounding Cultural Relativism'. *Anthropological Quarterly*. 80.3. (2007): 821–836. Print.

Rushdie, Salman. *The Satanic Verses*. London: Vintage, 1988. Print.

———. *The Moor's Last Sigh*. London: Vintage, 1997. Print.

Ruthven, Malise. *Fundamentalism: A Very Short Introduction*. Oxford: Oxford University Press, 2007. Print.

Scanlan, Margaret. 'Writers Among Terrorists: Don DeLillo's Mao II and the Rushdie Affair'. *Modern Fiction Studies*. 40.2. (1994): 229–252. Print.

Shryock, Andrew. *Islamophobia/Islamophilia: Beyond the Politics of Enemy and Friend*. Bloomington: Indiana University Press, 2010. Print.

Smith, Jay. 'Is the Qur'an the Word of God?' London: Hyde Park Christian Fellowship. 1996. Web. Accessed: 18 August 2010. <http://debate.org.uk/topics/history/debate/debate.html>.

Thatamanil, John J. 'Transreligious Theology as the Quest for Interreligious Wisdom: Defining, Defending, and Teaching Transreligious Theology'. *Open Theology*. 2. (2016): 354–362. Web. Accessed: 15 July 2018. <https://www.degruyter.com/downloadpdf/j/opth.2016.2.issue-1/opth-2016-0029/opth-2016-0029.pdf>.

Wildman, Wesley J. 'Theology Without Walls: The Future of Transreligious Theology'. *Open Theology*. 2. (2016): 242–247. Web. Accessed: 28 July 2018. <https://www.degruyter.com/downloadpdf/j/opth.2016.2.issue-1/opth-2016-0019/opth-2016-0019.pdf>.

Multimedia Sources

Apocrifu. Choreographed by Sidi Larbi Cherkaoui. 2007. Video Recording of Performance.

'Baby Love'. Performed by The Supremes. Written by Holland-Dozier-Holland. Motown Records. 1964. Song.

Foi. Choreographed by Sidi Larbi Cherkaoui. 2003. Video Recording of Performance.

Is The Qur'an Corrupted? Biblical Characters in the Qur'an. 2006. Web. Accessed: 17 August 2010. <http://www.youtube.com/watch?v=raw-SB7AjMo>.

'Somewhere Over the Rainbow'. Performed by Judy Garland. Written by Harold Arlen & Edgard Yipsel Harburg. Metro-Goldwyn-Mayer. 1939. Song.

Submission. Written by Ayaan Hirsi Ali. Produced by Theo Van Gogh. 2004. Film.

The Wizard of Oz. Directed by Victor Fleming. Metro-Goldwyn-Mayer. 1939. Film.

Interviews

Leboutte, Christine. Interview with author. London, June 2004.
Ómarsdóttir, Erna. Interview with author. London, June 2004.
Snellings, Dirk. Telephone interview with author. June 2004.

CHAPTER 5

Heteroglossia and Non-translation in *Myth*

Cherkaoui's works are filled with heteroglossic fragments of text that are not translated. The cross-cultural collaborative devising processes used by Cherkaoui are, to a certain extent, visible and audible in the staged work. In *Rien de Rien* (2000), stories in English, French, Russian and Slovakian are juxtaposed with a French chanson, an American pop song and a traditional African song. On the back wall, Arabic calligraphy provides a climbing frame for a dancer in a sacrilegious scene. A Francophone dancer spray-paints a slogan in Flemish. In *Foi* (2003), spectators are confronted with, for example, the Italian traditional song 'Passione de Guilianullo', Ars Nova songs in Latin, a travel story in French about a money-making scam in Martinique, the Icelandic lullaby 'Sofðu unga ástin mín', a nervous flirtation between a woman who speaks English and a man who speaks French, the Chinese song 'Qing Lang' and the Flemish song 'Ach Vlaendre Vrie'. In *zero degrees*, co-choreographed with Akram Khan, Cherkaoui sings the Hebrew song 'Yerushalayim Shel Zahav'. *Myth* (2007) features a militant, yet impenetrable, speech in Japanese. In *Babel^(words)* (co-choreographed with Damien Jalet, 2010), a group of dancers, lined up next to each other on their knees, exclaim the word 'land' in their native language, as they trace the space around them with their fingertips. Another scene from the work shows the performers profusely apologising to each other in different languages after a collision between the various aluminium cuboid frames designed by Antony Gormley. The apologies become more and more competitive and are transformed into a language

© The Author(s) 2019   131
L. Uytterhoeven, *Sidi Larbi Cherkaoui*, New World Choreographies,
https://doi.org/10.1007/978-3-030-27816-8_5

competition, in which the performers shout out tongue twisters in various languages. Each of these songs and utterances holds within it a depth of historical complexity in its cultural and sociopolitical significance.

Language plays an important role in the work of the Flemish-Moroccan Cherkaoui in a variety of ways. After growing up in a multilingual household in Belgium, Cherkaoui briefly embarked upon a translation studies course before choosing a career in dance performance and choreography. He entered the diverse transnational dance field in Flanders at the turn of the millennium, first studying at P.A.R.T.S, the contemporary dance school of Anne Teresa De Keersmaeker, and then performing and choreographing with Alain Platel's Les Ballets C. de la B., which, combined with his multilingual upbringing, may have prompted him to engage in a choreographic exploration of issues of speech and language in his work. These seem to be symptomatic of wider cultural issues for Cherkaoui. Therefore, theories of language, including translation studies, provide a useful lens through which to analyse the dramaturgical layers in his work and evaluate them in a broader cultural framework. In his complex dance theatre, texts are either spoken, sung or visually incorporated in the scenography in many different languages, including Dutch, French, English, Swedish, Slovakian, Portuguese, Japanese, Afrikaans and Arabic, largely without translation. These are the native languages of the performers, who are selected precisely because of their diverging cultural identities.

This chapter will include descriptive analysis of the highly complex work *Myth* to illustrate how Cherkaoui incorporates languages in his dance works and to evaluate possible cultural implications of his theatrical practice for spectators. This chapter will engage in detailed analysis of the dramaturgical implications of Cherkaoui's decision not to translate languages. First, however, it is useful to map out theatre scholar Marvin Carlson's discussion of heteroglossic theatre practices, particularly as they relate to Flanders, in more detail, and to consider the implications of Cherkaoui's work in relation to the emerging argument that heteroglossic theatre holds the potential to counter nationalism.

Mapping Heteroglossic Theatre in Flanders

Carlson considers heteroglossic theatre to be exemplary of a kind of postmodern language play aiming to destabilise established monoglossic theatrical traditions and, with Hans-Thies Lehmann and his framework of postdramatic theatre, the notion of the stable dramatic text itself. Cherkaoui's dance theatre significantly differs from text-based theatre practices, as it neither emerges from a dramatic text nor aims directly to uproot the text through the strategies identified by Lehmann and Carlson; the dramatic text is irrelevant to Cherkaoui's work. Nevertheless, the developments in European, and more specifically Flemish, theatre described by Carlson and Lehmann form part of the wider artistic context in which Cherkaoui came of age as a performer and choreographer and are hence worth briefly exploring here.

While Cherkaoui's works can easily be seen to fit with Carlson's framework of heteroglossic language play, I will argue in this chapter that they present a further and direct challenge, which Carlson's model does not account for. With Carlson, the inclusion of a multiplicity of languages in Cherkaoui's works could be read as an opposing of the nationalism implicit in some traditional monoglossic theatre. Monoglossia, however, does not characterise the Flemish theatre and dance landscape around the turn of the millennium, when Cherkaoui began to create work, at all. Therefore, he can be considered to be not alone in resisting nationalism through a rejection of theatrical monoglossia. Carlson highlights, for example, De Keersmaeker's exploration of fragments of texts by Dostoyevsky, Tolstoy, Brecht and Handke, recited in different languages as postmodern 'linguistic collage' (172). Other examples presented by Carlson include Needcompany's *King Lear* (2001), in which languages are deliberately mixed as a joke, and Tom Lanoye and Luk Perceval's *Schlachten!* (1999). In the latter, English and Flemish (or German for the performances in Germany and Austria) versions of Shakespeare's *Richard II* and *Richard III* are sliced up and alternated or 'interpenetrated' (Carlson 176). The language used gradually descends from classical and stately old Flemish, German and French into an American slang imitating Tarantino films and Motown. Lanoye explained that the English used at the end of the play represents 'the confusion of languages that surrounds us today', suggesting that 'we live in a speech aquarium, which seems, depending on how you view it, extremely rich and varied or extremely polluted' (Lanoye cited in Carlson 178).

Whereas Carlson's examples are concerned with (re)-staging existing texts or plays, Cherkaoui's works sit firmly outside the dramatic tradition, or even the postdramatic echoes thereof. These theatre makers are concerned with vastly different material to that of Cherkaoui. For example, to illustrate the difference in artistic concerns between these artists and Cherkaoui, Jan Lauwers of Needcompany explains that he 'sought a non-dramatic text that he could "construct" on stage, instead of being reduced to the rather dissatisfying role of the director and staging an already created work' (qtd. in Lehmann 108). Lehmann considers Lauwers to produce 'postepic narration' (108) and 'scenic poems' (111). Cherkaoui, in contrast, rarely works with full-length existing written texts, especially dramatic texts, opting for informal storytelling, orally transmitted stories and songs, and fragments of texts written by the performers. This privileging of oral traditions can be seen as challenging the power of the written word in, for example, mainstream history in *Myth* or religious fundamentalism in *Apocrifu* (2007).

What sets Cherkaoui's work further apart from the fin-de-millennium works highlighted by Carlson, is that the languages that are featured in Carlson's examples are mainly limited to European languages. Given that a large portion of Flemish people routinely speak French, English and German, this limited postmodern language play does not challenge the cultural bias of multilingual Flemish theatregoers as fully as Cherkaoui's work does. He, significantly, mixes languages that are perhaps less prevalent in the Flemish cultural consciousness at the turn of the millennium, such as Russian, Slovenian, Arabic, Icelandic, Japanese and Hebrew. Nevertheless, Carlson's conclusion that these artists allow 'material, including language, from different cultures to play against material from other cultures, without necessarily privileging any particular cultural material, even that most familiar to a presumed majority of the audience' (179) holds some validity for Cherkaoui's work. Indeed, while Carlson typifies this, perhaps prematurely, as 'a fugal chorus of voices, in some cases with none of them claiming linguistic primacy, weaving new theatrical mixtures for the audiences of a new multicultural society' (179), despite its strong Western European cultural bias, it will be argued in this chapter that Cherkaoui's work aligns itself with transculturalism even more strongly and makes a decisive intervention in debates surrounding language and culture.

In late twentieth-century Belgium where Cherkaoui grew up, language was a sore point and continues to be so, as demonstrated by the political impasse from 2007 to 2011 between Flemish and Walloon parties in the extended process of government formation, discussed at length in the introductory Chapter 1. Nationalism is tied to xenophobia in the context of the populist radical right. I argue that Cherkaoui's heteroglossic dramaturgy exceeds the potential of heteroglossic theatre to oppose nationalism ascribed to it by Carlson. This more far-reaching potential to elicit change in audiences' perceptions of language and culture lies in his resolute choice for non-translation, as will be explored through analysis of *Myth* in the following section.

Non-translation in *Myth*

Salient examples of non-translation can be found in *Myth*, the first large-scale production Cherkaoui made as artist in residence at the Antwerp Toneelhuis in collaboration with Patrizia Bovi's Ensemble Micrologus, which specialises in vocal and instrumental medieval music of the Mediterranean region. *Myth* is a multi-layered, polyglot work, in which the production of meaning is highly complicated and requires a specific kind of dramaturgical labour from the spectator. In this section, it will be argued that the choreographer's creative methodology entailed, on this occasion, the physical, musical, textual and visual exploration of myth as a central theme by a wide range of culturally diverse performers. As demonstrated in Chapter 3, the seeking out of performers who have interesting vocal or corporeal stories to tell—stories of displacement through migration or mixedness—can be considered representative of Cherkaoui's practice. The production brought together twenty-one performers on stage. After a sustained period of international touring and collaborations abroad, *Myth* marked Cherkaoui's albeit temporary, return to his home town, Antwerp. Apart from Bovi and her Ensemble Micrologus and dramaturg Guy Cools, Cherkaoui also collaborated with choreography assistant Nienke Reehorst, a former dancer with Wim Vandekeybus's Ultima Vez, who co-choreographed *Ook* (2002) with Cherkaoui for Theater Stap, a theatre company working with actors with learning disabilities.

In this section, I will introduce *Myth* as a work with an emphasis on the use of language and heteroglossia. For further analysis of the work, please read this chapter in conjunction with Chapter 6, in which I discuss the religious and psychoanalytical layers of the work from a more choreographic point of view, including the Jungian imagery created by Cherkaoui. *Myth* is labelled by Cherkaoui as the second part of a trilogy, *Foi* being the first part and *Babel(words)* being the final part. We see a number of performers recurring in the works in this trilogy. *Myth* begins with a slow and silent scene of flirtation and rejection, played by Marc Wagemans and Ann Dockx, who both have Down's syndrome and whom Cherkaoui met while he worked with Theater Stap when he created *Ook*. Wagemans was also part of the cast for *Foi*, so his presence in *Myth* is a continuation. Others from the cast of *Foi* can also be recognised in *Myth*: Christine Leboutte, Ulrika Kinn Svensson and Darryl E. Woods are some of the other protagonists, while Alexandra Gilbert and Jalet are recurring presences in the chorus.

The chorus in *Myth* takes the form of a troupe of shadow figures, dressed entirely in black and moving with and around the protagonists by sliding on the floor as they walk. Sometimes the shadows react neutrally to the protagonists' movements, but increasingly they interfere in a way that haunts and taunts the protagonists, and eventually also manipulates their actions. Examples of this are analysed in further detail in Chapter 6. Woods is haunted by his shadows, as they play tricks on him and deliberately set out to scare him.

There are several instances of the characters in *Myth* talking over and next to one another in different languages, exemplifying polyglossia. For example, Gilbert wears a long black wig in which her toes are stuck and performs contorted movements, resembling a furry creature. Svensson utters mutterings in disgust at this furry 'animal' in Swedish. She walks over to Gilbert, puts on gloves and forcible pushes her down, as if crushing this 'vermin', bringing the idyllic harp music to an abrupt end. Svensson emphatically exclaims the word 'asthma', while she twists Gilbert's limbs, pulls her by the hair, kicks her and bends her over backwards, then places her foot on Gilbert's pelvis and pushes her down flat, to horrified gasps in the audience. Svensson drags Gilbert away. Before finally sitting down, however, Svensson cannot resist but drape a scarf made of the furs of several animals around her neck, in a hugely ironic gesture, which elicits laughs from the audience. Svensson tells Dockx, in Flemish: 'Please go and do some dusting!', to which Dockx gets up and walks over to the bookshelf, a duster in hand.

Later, Peter Jaško pursues Bouche, trying to embrace her, but she slips away. He shouts at her in Slovakian. He then attempts to kiss her, but Dockx breaks them up by smashing her fan down onto their hands and shouting 'Enough!'. Wagemans loudly cries 'Nee!', meaning 'no' in Dutch. In the middle of the work, after a harrowing scene in which Woods hurls insensitive comments at her, Dockx sings the traditional, sixteenth-century, Flemish song 'Ick seg adieu', *a capella*. The lyrics translate as 'I bid adieu. The two of us, we must part. Until the next time we meet, I will long for your comfort. I leave my heart with you, for where you are, I shall also be. In joy or grief, always shall I be yours with all my heart' (Camerata Trajectina). Then, Leboutte, accompanied by the lute, fiddle, and flute, sings the same song again. Other voices join in and harmonise.

In the middle of *Myth*, Leboutte and Dockx sit together and begin a conversation across languages, where Leboutte elaborately expresses her feelings in French and Dockx responds with one-liners in Flemish, offering life advice, for example, 'Life doesn't change; what matters is how you perceive it' and 'That is not self-evident'. Dockx utters the phrase 'Raar maar waar' which translates as 'Weird, but true' and is often used to affirm surprising, fun facts. Despite speaking different languages, Leboutte keeps fuelling the conversation with more memories. Dockx finishes the conversation by insisting that she really is not a pessimist.

Towards the end of *Myth*, there is a scene that is most relevant to the theme of non-translation, notably, a lengthy Japanese speech that goes without translation, which is the main focus of this chapter. In the build-up to Satoshi Kudo's reciting of this Japanese text, Svensson recites Carl Gustav Jung's text 'The Christ Within' (Jung *Symbolic Life* 280), proclaiming how Christ is within each person, equating the figure of Christ to the potential of the Self within each human being waiting to be realised. A transcription and further discussion of this text can be found in Chapter 6. Wagemans has knelt down to kiss her hand, despite being lectured at pedantically by Svensson. She puts a leash around his neck before pushing him on his hands and knees, leading him around the stage, and putting one of her feet on his back; she then rests her elbow on her knee, takes off her glasses and faces the audience reciting Jung's writing. The sound of Svensson's voice is drowned out by the percussive song *Brumas e mors*. The translation from Latin to English is: 'Man, bewail! Flee, flee, these mortal things. Why do you love the transient? All are dreams, they pass and return not. The world, the flesh, the Devil, money saw in men this hatred: Discord, and not Concord rules, along with Avarice too; Simon is judge in the Church. Listen to this written example: Brumas is death! O wretched man! You are never stable. How can you be joyful? Your life is frail and your death is lamentable; why then, are you not in mourning? For you must go in death, never to return. Fragile as ice, tomorrow you must die. Your lot in this life is to die but once; therefore, be assured and do not doubt: Brumas is death! O, alas what peril!' (Micrologus) The word 'Brumas' in the title is left untranslated. It may be derived from the Latin word 'bruma', referring to the winter solstice, the shortest day of the year, as an abbreviation of the superlative 'brevissima'. However, in Spanish, the word 'bruma' means mist, and the idea of 'las brumas' or 'the mists' has been tied to the waters surrounding Hades, the Greek god of the underworld (Faszer-McMahon 169).

The physical subordination and social humiliation of Wagemans are pushed to the extreme. Svensson has tied the leash to the double doors and demands that Wagemans shares his opinion about the Jung text she has just finished reciting. 'Tell me, what is your opinion? Huh? I'm giving you the space here to share your thoughts. So, tell me...' Leboutte interrupts her, in French, saying that she is right and that it is important to give Wagemans a voice that he has a right to be heard. Svensson retorts, full of disdain: 'I don't speak French'. Sri Louise jumps into the discussion, trying to bring the conversation back to the transcultural elements Jung introduces in his text: 'Well, yes, from a Vedantic standpoint, the Atman is already a sinless reality'. Svensson interrupts her: 'Well, I didn't ask for your opinion, did I?' Leboutte talks French. Svensson barks back at her: 'I'm not talking to you!'. Louise says: 'I agree, quite frankly, modern psychology will never be able to resolve the basic existential crisis'. 'I'm talking to him', Svensson says, pointing down at Wagemans. Woods asks: 'I'm sorry, could you repeat the part about the At-man? [making it rhyme with Batman] I missed that bit...' Leboutte replies: 'Je pense que... [I think that...]' and she and Louise talk emphatically over each other. Svensson drags Wagemans to his feet. She shouts: 'Stop it!' Woods still keeps going: 'Well, my analyst tells me that...'. Svensson insists: 'Shut up! [then at Wagemans] Tell them, what is your opinion? Now!' She punches his shoulder (Fig. 5.1).

Wagemans snatches Svensson's glasses off her face and puts them on. He points his index finger right in her face. Kudo has slowly slipped through a trapdoor in the back wall and stands behind Svensson. He performs a monologue, speaking rapidly and loudly in Japanese. Wagemans repeatedly takes his finger away and points it back in Svensson's face. It is as if he is speaking, not Kudo. Leboutte and Louise look on in puzzlement. Louise quietly giggles at the absurdity of the scene. Slowly Kudo slides over to stand behind Wagemans instead.

In a conversation with Kudo after my first viewing of the work, I asked him what he was saying and he explained: 'it's the history of the Second World War from a Japanese point of view' (Kudo). Months later, after I had become more and more intrigued by this scene in subsequent viewings, he and I sat down to translate the Japanese text into English. We worked our way through the text word for word. Kudo listened to

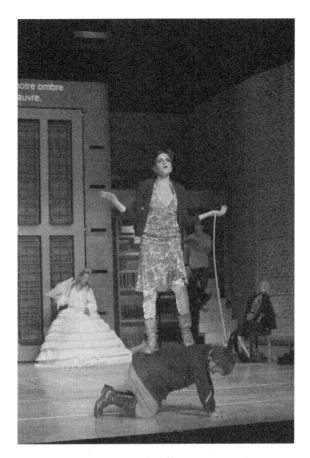

Fig. 5.1 Ulrika Kinn Svensson and Marc Wagemans in *Myth* (Photo by Laurent Philippe)

his own speech as part of a video recording of the performance, played on his laptop, using in-ear headphones, pausing after every little phrase. I wrote down Kudo's translation in my notebook. The text was far more provocative than I had anticipated:

> Do you know why Japan was attacked by the atomic bomb? [...] Do you know how many people were victims of these atomic bombs? [...] 270.000 people became victims, just because you wanted to experiment with the

atomic bomb; just because you wanted to show your power to Russia and Germany. [...] But you just said that you saved Asia from Japan. [...] What did you say after the Second World War? No more Hiroshima. And it was a lie. The depleted uranium bombs you used in the Gulf War were nuclear weapons! [...] And finally, in 2001, the revenge started. On September 11th the New York World Trade Center was destroyed. That day, on television, CNN showed you crying and trying to escape. They showed how scared you are. Yes, and you finally got it: the rights of the victim. And do you believe that if you are a victim, you are forgiven by God? And in 2003, you had a perfect excuse: you started another war, Iraq War. But your own citizens died in this war. And now you say you are a victim of George Bush, who was chosen by the people for the people. [...] I know you are not a victim. [...] (Kudo)

During the creation process, Cherkaoui had given Kudo the task to write a text about trauma in his native language, focusing on the performers' personal perspectives and experiences in a transcultural bid to find elements that bind people together beyond cultural difference. Initially, Kudo purely outlined historical facts, listing dates and events, but the scene in which it was included inspired him to add his emotional response as well. The Japanese text follows a scene in which Wagemans, a performer with Down's syndrome, is singled out, physically subordinated, humiliated and exposed in his inability to express himself verbally. The change of voice and tone is the result of Kudo's creative process in engaging with the dramaturgical context of the scene. Kudo's text can be understood as an amplification of repressed Japanese feelings of injustice and trauma which have been written out of mainstream historical discourse. It is juxtaposed to Wagemans's fierce, repetitive and rhythmical finger-pointing towards his aggressors. Similarities between the two performers' frustrations bubble towards the dramaturgical surface after researching and seeking translation of the Japanese text. The dramaturgical labour in which I engaged as a spectator after the performance allowed me to access another layer of meaning in the work, but it was left to my own initiative to pursue my curiosity and engage in cross-cultural dialogue with Kudo. Without the translation, the sense of powerlessness is not conveyed any less strongly by the non-verbal content of the scene alone, but the spectator's response remains affective rather than conscious, and the understanding of the complex dramaturgical layers present in the work limited.

A DRAMATURGY OF NON-TRANSLATION
AS POSTCOLONIAL CRITIQUE

In general, when discussing Cherkaoui's work, because texts are not translated, spectators who may not know the array of languages spoken, sung or written, are left to their own devices to 'make sense' of their function in the overarching dramaturgy of the works. This resolute act of non-translation problematises, and even undermines, the signification process. Meaning appears hidden to the spectator, who is incapable of accessing it. As in postdramatic theatre, the spectators' desire to understand is frustrated and, with the performers, they become part of a 'shared space of language problems' (Lehmann 147). This practice challenges the concept of dramaturgy as mediation between artist and audience, anticipating audiences' perception in relation to the artist's intended meaning (Turner & Behrndt 101 and 156). A rejection of the role of translator implies a rejection of authorial responsibility for meaning-making. In this sense, Cherkaoui's dramaturgy of non-translation aligns itself with the Flemish discourse on new dramaturgies at the turn of the millennium, which refuses the legitimising function of dramaturgy as embodied in the figure of the dramaturg (Van Kerkhoven; Van Imschoot; De Vuyst). Van Imschoot expressed a certain anxiety about the allocation of language and discourse to the realm of the dramaturg, as this may indicate in some instances that the dramaturg compensates for a perceived lack of knowledge or intellectual capacity. De Vuyst considers dramaturgy to fulfil a legitimising and didactic role, and therefore the dramaturg to embody a perceived shortcoming. A solution to the perceived power imbalances inherent in the choreographer-dramaturg relationship adopted by Cherkaoui is to share the dramaturgical function between all the artistic collaborators rather than singling out this responsibility in the sole figure of the professional dramaturg. In addition to this shared dramaturgy, he invites a range of dramaturgical interlocutors to the creative process: friends, friends of friends, visitors and outsiders. In a broader sense, I argue that the dramaturgical process extends beyond the creation of the work to include the performance and the work's relationship with spectators, who are invited to engage in further macro-dramaturgical dialogue about the work with cultural others and, among other transcultural aspects, the texts spoken in languages that were inaccessible during the performance itself.

In the light of the politics of translation within postcolonialism, Cherkaoui rejects the burden of responsibility for translation, which is often put on the Other, the immigrant, to translate for the benefit of the dominant culture. Likewise, in recent years, translation scholars have emphasised the limitations of translation (Bassnett & Lefevere; Spivak; Venuti). For the purposes of this chapter, Lawrence Venuti's discussion of the contrasting translation practices of 'domestication' and 'foreignizing' provides a useful entry point into the existing postcolonial critiques of translation. On the one hand, domesticating translation practices are considered 'ethnocentric' and, on the other, foreignising translations are seen to be 'ethnodeviant' acts of resistance against racist and imperialist outlooks (Venuti *Translation Studies* 15). However, translation scholars tend to agree that no translation can grant the reader unmediated access to the foreign (Berman; Venuti; Bassnett & Trivedi). Venuti's concept of 'foreignizing' implies a drawing attention to the act of translation through playful and rebellious translations which cannot become invisible and therefore cannot uphold the illusion inherent in 'domestication'. Undertaking a historiographical and genealogical approach to mapping the history of English language translation, Venuti (*Translator's Invisibility*) undermines the notion of fluency in translation which dominates the canons of accuracy, and rather sees this generally accepted emphasis on fluency as culturally specific and historically determined. Taking into account ethical concerns towards other languages and cultures, Venuti further develops Schleiermacher's concept of 'domestication' in translation referring to its emphasis on fluency. He argues that

> British and American publishers [...] have reaped the financial benefits of successfully imposing English-language cultural values on a vast foreign readership, while producing cultures that are aggressively monolingual, unreceptive to foreign literatures, accustomed to fluent translations that invisibly inscribe foreign texts with British and American values and provide readers with the narcissistic experience of recognizing their own culture in a cultural other. (Venuti *Translator's Invisibility* 12)

He also extends this concept from translation practices to 'British and American relations with cultural others', which he sees as characterised by 'a complacency that can be described – without too much exaggeration – as imperialistic abroad and xenophobic at home' (Venuti *Translator's Invisibility* 13).

Cherkaoui and co-choreographer Jalet provide an interesting chore-ographic commentary on this British and American approach to other cultures in *Babel$^{(words)}$*, another production made for the Antwerp Toneelhuis, which becomes the focus of discussion in Chapter 7. In an ironic scene, performer Darryl E. Woods lists the virtues and benefits of the English language as 'the greatest language on earth' in an over-the-top, arrogant manner:

> English is the most widespread language in the world and is more widely spoken and written than any other language. Over 400 million people use the English vocabulary as a mother tongue, only surpassed in numbers, but not in distribution by speakers of the many varieties of Chinese. Over 700 million people, speak English, as a foreign language. [...] English is the medium for 80% of the information stored in the world's computers. [...] No language has more synonyms than English. People who count English as their mother tongue make up less than 10% of the world's pop-ulation, but possess over 30% of the world's economic power. Therefore, in terms of the quantity of transmitted information, English is the leader by far.

All the while, he treads, sits and reclines on the human furniture that is made up by the other non-native English speaking performers, to illus-trate the destructive powers of this kind of lingering imperialism. In *Babel$^{(words)}$*, Cherkaoui and Jalet can be seen to stage a theatrical response to the issues that translation theorists are identifying.

Examining these debates in more detail, for Venuti, foreignising trans-lations can be 'a form of resistance against ethnocentrism and racism, cultural narcissism and imperialism' (Venuti *Translator's Invisibility* 16), as they 'tend to flaunt their partiality [in the process of interpreting the foreign text] instead of concealing it' (Venuti *Translator's Invisibility* 28–29). Inevitably, 'in an effort to do right abroad, this translation prac-tice must do wrong at home [...] stag[ing] an alien reading experience' (Venuti *Translator's Invisibility* 15–16). However, for Cherkaoui, rather than foreignising, opting not to translate is a valid and powerful choice available to him, which echoes Venuti's critique of domesticating trans-lation, and the absence of translation precisely highlights the political problems inherent in translation.

These problems were already highlighted by Benjamin in his essay 'The Task of the Translator', which was first published in 1923 as an introduction to his own translation of the poetry by Baudelaire.

The concerns raised by Benjamin are shared by current translation scholars, such as Susan Bassnett, Gayatri Chakravorty Spivak and Venuti, the
latter of whom included the essay as the opening text in his *Translation
Studies Reader*, and are valuable to the examination of Cherkaoui's
theatrical practice of non-translation. Quoting the translator and poet
Pannwitz, and echoing Schleiermacher, Benjamin offers a resolute critique on domestication:

> Our translations, even the best ones, proceed from a wrong premise.
> They want to turn Hindi, Greek, English into German instead of turning
> German into Hindi, Greek, English. Our translators have a far greater rev-
> erence for the usage of their own language than for the spirit of the foreign
> works. [...] The basic error of the translator is that he preserves the state in
> which his own language happens to be instead of allowing his language to
> be powerfully affected by the foreign tongue. (Benjamin 'Task' 22)

Although other parts of Benjamin's text seem devoid of cultural concerns and focus instead on religion and philosophy, this rejection of
domestication is strongly in line with current thought in translation studies, as is the advocating of foreignising. Benjamin emphasises a complete
disregard of the needs of the reader, or an 'ideal' receiver. One should
not read a translation for meaning, but through translation one can
aspire to 'pure language', the language of God as opposed to 'inadequate human languages', preceding the event of Babel (Benjamin 'Task'
17). Pure language is 'free of meaning', and attained through revealing
in the translation 'how the "mutually exclusive" differences among languages coexist with "complementary" intentions to communicate and to
refer, intentions that are derailed by the differences, because differences
between source and target language are exposed' (Venuti *Translation
Studies* 11). The aim of translation, for Benjamin, is therefore not to produce an accurate, fluent or seemingly neutral version of the original text.
Translation has to stay as close to the original as possible in syntax and
way of expressing things, and not try to transfer meaning, even if this is
at the cost of aesthetic aspects (Dudek).

> The pure language is released in the translation through literalism, espe-
> cially in syntax, which result in departures from current standard usage.
> Benjamin is reviving Schleiermacher's notion of foreignizing translation,
> wherein the reader of the translated text is brought as close as possible to

the foreign one through close renderings that transform the translating language. (Venuti *Translation Studies* 11–12)

Dudek notes that the idea of untranslatability is sometimes associated with Benjamin's essay. 'This view is often taken by referring to the ambiguity of the title: the German title "Die Aufgabe des Übersetzers" could also be translated as "The Surrender of the Translator"' (Dudek). Cherkaoui, by refusing to translate, can be considered to surrender and dissociate himself in his work from translation practices which are ethnocentric and serve an imperial, colonising attitude towards other cultural practices. Even if it is not through translation practices, as Benjamin suggests, Cherkaoui is concerned with emphasising cultural difference in his choreographies. Instead, he can be seen to openly resist translation practices as a methodology.

What does it mean for Cherkaoui to renounce the burden of responsibility of translation, which is often put on the Other, the immigrant, to translate for the benefit of the dominant culture? Welcker posits that 'Colonial translation is a one-way exchange, a toll of the dominant culture to assimilate myths and histories of the colonized culture and altering customs, phrases and intent so that these stories fit within the recognized confines of the "new" culture'. As a postcolonial figure and a xenophile, Cherkaoui refuses to translate for the benefit of merely Western audiences. Alternative, postcolonial voices are embraced in his works, but the key to accessing their message is placed in the hands of the spectator. The absence of translation precisely highlights, firstly, the jarring need for translation and, secondly, the political problems of translation.

The literary theorist and feminist critic Spivak, discussing the politics of translation, criticises the impulse of some feminists to focus on the idea that women across cultures have something in common. She argues that this kind of women's solidarity is only the first step, but that learning the woman's mother-tongue is the second step. Sharing a language means sharing a world view, or how one makes sense of things, and serves as a 'preparation for the intimacy of cultural translation' (Spivak 192). Spivak asserts that 'if you are interested in talking about the other, and/or in making a claim to be the other, it is crucial to learn other languages' (192). Cherkaoui bypasses the function of translation, which tends to mask the fact that we cannot ever understand the Other, and instead resolutely draws attention to the fact that spectator and performer (most probably) do not share the same language. Without translation, the spectator is prevented from laying claim to the Other as promised by domesticating translation practices, even in the name of solidarity.

Paradoxically, while compromising the conventional mode of communication based on a shared language, Cherkaoui actually aims to improve the understanding between people of different cultural backgrounds through his choreography (Olaerts 17). He acknowledges, however, that this is utopian. Nonetheless, he was recognised for this aim by UNESCO in April 2011, when he was honoured for promoting dialogue across cultures. Likewise, Venuti imagines that foreignising translation may help to 'establish more democratic cultural exchanges' and 'change receiving cultural values' (*Translator's Invisibility* 34). Cherkaoui's choice of non-translation and his revealing of the jarring need for translation in the performance situation can therefore be seen as preceding Spivak's first step of working towards the intimacy of cultural translation, so that performers and spectators may begin to share their various world views. The working towards bridging the gaps left by Cherkaoui's non-translation, by having cross-cultural conversations with others after the performance moment, forms part of the continuous dramaturgy of the spectator.

Cherkaoui's dramaturgy of non-translation problematises, and even undermines, the signification process, as meaning appears hidden to the spectators, who are left to their own devices to 'make sense' of the performance. Likewise, Cherkaoui's practice challenges the notion of dramaturgy as mediation between artist and audience (Turner & Behrndt). His deliberate dramaturgies of non-translation give rise to the continuous macro dramaturgy of the spectator, as he invites spectators to feel, appreciate, respond to and reflect on, what it is like to experience the jarring need for translation and to be between cultures, histories and identities. The labour that he invites spectators to engage in may entail conversations with cultural others after the performance moment to explore the transcultural networks of various dramaturgical layers. The paradox of Cherkaoui's dramaturgies lies in the fact that he translates, guides and explains less, in order for spectators to begin to understand more through their own continuous dramaturgical work.

However, it is important to caution against simply extending the non-translation argument to dance. In a rather twee scene in the middle of *Myth*, Jaško and Milan Herich perform a series of heel-clicking movements and footwork patterns from Slovakian folk dance. Drums, trumpets, bagpipes and castanets constitute the musical landscape, and the rhythmical folk dancing is juxtaposed with Woods launching into a Hollywood-style tap dance, holding a small, round mirror in one hand. A spotlight is on Woods centre stage, with Jaško and Herich moving in the periphery of the light, and behind them three other dancers perform another upbeat folk dance in semi-darkness. Suddenly the music stops and the spotlight disappears while the whole stage is lit up entirely again. Woods performs a tap shuffle step travelling sideways, still looking in the mirror, not looking at where he is going, then trips over another dancer and a bench, falling flat on the floor. Dockx, who has been watching him all along, exclaims an ironic 'wow' and performs a giggling gesture with her shoulders.

The scene is upbeat, light and celebratory in tone. It caused a sense of unease with me because of the easy, uncomplicated juxtaposition of dances from different cultures to the extent that this layering emphasises what the dance forms share in common while almost erasing the differences. Hence, dance is presented as universal as it transcends culture and the verbal and can supposedly be understood by people across cultures. The ending of the scene brings the relief of irony, suggesting that this easy, physical connection across culture through dance is a laughable fantasy. Contrast this to the painstaking attempts at transcultural transformation Cherkaoui subjected himself to in *zero degrees*, *Dunas* and *Play*, discussed in Chapter 3, each with varying degrees of what critics perceived as 'success'. Cherkaoui tried and ultimately failed to take on the ways of moving of the others, his dancing partners Khan, Pagés and Shivalingappa. The dramaturgy worked in such a way that spectators could tell the difference in execution of the movement; they could tell that Cherkaoui was not a native 'speaker' of this other dance language. In effect, this choreographic process resembles the foreignising translation practices mentioned above. However, such a gap does not tend to exist in the spectator's engagement when watching culturally specific dance when it is presented without a dramaturgical strategy to raise questions, such as a dance partner who did not achieve fluency in that way of moving or self-effacing irony. I am therefore concerned that the argument about non-translation of languages as a dramaturgical device to resist a dominant Western world view should not be extended to the inclusion of 'culturally different' dance material. In contrast to the exclusion caused by an inability to speak a language that is spoken on stage and left untranslated, the same barriers do not exist with dance. The colonising reflex of Western audiences to consume, appropriate and possess other dance forms may simply be too strong.

BIBLIOGRAPHY

Bassnett, Susan & Lefevere, André. *Translation, History, and Culture*. London and New York: Pinter Publishers, 1990. Print.

Bassnett, Susan & Trivedi, Harish. *Postcolonial Translation: Theory and Practice*. London: Routledge, 1999. Print.

Benjamin, Walter. *Illuminations*. New York: Schocken Books, 1968. Print.

———. (trans. Harry Zohn) 'The Task of the Translator: An Introduction to the Translation of Baudelaire's *Tableaus Parisiens*'. *Translation Studies Reader*. Ed. Venuti, Lawrence. Florence, NY: Routledge, 1999. 15–25. Print.

Berman, Antoine. *The Experience of the Foreign: Culture and Translation in Romantic Germany*. Albany: State University of New York Press, 1992. Print.

Carlson, Marvin. *Speaking in Tongues: Language at Play in the Theatre*. Ann Arbor: The University of Michigan Press, 2006. Print.

De Vuyst, Hildegard. 'Een Dramaturgie Van Het Gebrek: Paradoxen en Dubbelzinnigheden'. *Etcetera*. 17.68. (1999): 65–66. Print.

Dudek, Sarah. 'Walter Benjamin & the Religion of Translation'. *Cipher Journal*. Web. Accessed: 29 March 2011. <http://www.cipherjournal.com/html/dudek_benjamin.html>.

Faszer-McMahon, Debra. *Cultural Encounters in Contemporary Spain: The Poetry of Clara Janés*. Lewisburg, PA: Bucknell University Press, 2010. Print.

Jung, Carl Gustav. (trans. R.F.C. Hull) *The Symbolic Life: Miscellaneous Writings*. London: Routledge and Kegan Paul, 1977. Print.

Kudo, Satoshi. Original Japanese text cited in *Myth*, translated by Kudo, Antwerp, May 2009.

Lehmann, Hans-Thies. (trans. Karen Juers-Munby) *Postdramatic Theatre*. London: Routledge. 2006. Print.

Micrologus. *Myth—Sidi Larbi Cherkaoui: The Music*. 2007. Booklet with CD.

Olaerts, An. 'Marokkaan uit Hoboken én Choreograaf van het Jaar'. *Vacature*. 31 October 2008. 14–17. Print.

Spivak, Gayatri Chakravorty. *Outside in the Teaching Machine*. London: Routledge, 1993. Print.

Turner, Cathy & Behrndt, Synne. *Dramaturgy and Performance*. Basingstoke: Palgrave Macmillan, 2008. Print.

Van Imschoot, Myriam. 'Anxious Dramaturgy'. *Women & Performance: A Journal of Feminist Theory*. 26.13:2. (2003): 57–68. Print.

Van Kerkhoven, Marianne. 'Looking Without Pencil in the Hand'. *Theaterschrift*. 5–6. (1994): 140–148. Print.

———. 'Van de Kleine en Grote Dramaturgie: Pleidooi voor een "Interlocuteur"'. *Etcetera*. 17.68. (1999): 67–69. Print.

———. 'European Dramaturgy in the 21st Century'. *Performance Research*. 14.3. (2009): 7–11. Print.

Venuti, Lawrence. Ed. *Translation Studies Reader.* Florence, KY: Routledge, 1999. Print.

———. *The Translator's Invisibility: A History of Translation.* 2nd Ed. London: Routledge, 2008. Print.

Welcker, Ellen. 'Only Poems Can Translate Poems: On the Impossibility and Necessity of Translation'. *The Quarterly Conversation.* 2008. Web. Accessed: 23 July 2010. <http://quarterlyconversation.com/only-poems-can-translate-poems-on-the-impossibility-and-necessity-of-translation>.

Multimedia Source

Myth. Choreographed by Sidi Larbi Cherkaoui. 2007. Video Recording of Performance.

CHAPTER 6

Dreamwork, Circumambulation and Engaged Spectatorship in *Myth*

In *Myth* (2007), Cherkaoui posits religion as a kind of myth. As explored in Chapter 4, religion is a recurring theme for Cherkaoui, who was raised both Muslim and Catholic. *Myth* features a range of elements from Christian theology and mysticism, for example, notions of purgatory, sin, crucifixion and salvation. When the work begins, the dramaturgical emphasis is on the act of waiting. The opening scene sees six protagonists sitting on benches and chairs at the edges of the stage space, which is filled with leather-bound books on shelves as in a library. The space is dominated by an imposing double door in the back wall, stage left. A Flemish translation of a Chinese proverb is projected above the double doors: 'Voor wie weet te wachten, opent de tijd zijn deuren' ('For those who know how to wait, time opens its doors'). Perhaps this is a waiting room? If so, some people have been waiting a long time indeed, I realise, as my eyes are drawn towards a skeleton on a chair. Patrizia Bovi's Ensemble Micrologus initiates the medieval song 'Crucifixum in carne', evoking the crucifixion of Jesus Christ, with a rolling pattern of the goblet drum. This place that the protagonists find themselves in could be purgatory, which in Roman Catholic theology refers to a process of purification for those whose sins are forgivable but require temporary punishment, before they are permitted into heaven.

The medieval and traditional music, performed by Ensemble Micrologus and Cherkaoui's longstanding collaborators Christine Leboutte and Damien Jalet, emerges from a range of Christian practices of worship and addresses notions of the Holy Virgin, pilgrimage and the

© The Author(s) 2019
L. Uytterhoeven, *Sidi Larbi Cherkaoui*, New World Choreographies,
https://doi.org/10.1007/978-3-030-27816-8_6

resurrection of Christ. At the start of the work, Leboutte embarks on the 'Gospin plač', a passion song from the fifteenth century performed on the Croatian island of Hvar as part of a night procession on Maundy Thursday, the Thursday before Easter. Jalet also joins in with the singing. The song is octosyllabic, meaning it consists of only eight syllables; however, Leboutte and Jalet linger with each syllable as the piercing sounds descend and ascend on an unusual scale, exploring the tensions arising from the tonal intervals until the melody finds resolution on a comforting note. Later, the soothing tones of the harp and Bovi's voice emerge in the Iberian cantiga 'Běeito foi o dia', which praises the moment of the birth of the Virgin Mary. In the middle of *Myth*, Sri Louise and James O'Hara, both dressed in black, approach each other centre stage and dance a virtuoso duet together, to the *a capella* song 'Salve Regina', which the whole cast harmonises together. The text of the song translates as: 'Hail, Queen of mercy, the life and sweetness of every believer, our hope and fount of harmony' (Micrologus). Louise and O'Hara connect their hands and lean, slide, spin, roll and lift each other, all the while maintaining that touch of their hands on each other's bodies. Towards the end of the work, Bovi sings the Sephardic traditional song 'Mas ariva' *a capella* to accompany a duet between Ann Dockx and Louise.

However, illustrating Cherkaoui's transreligious approach, secular songs are also included, dealing with transcendental and natural themes, such as the stars, the waves of the sea and love. Bovi and Jalet, standing on a ridge up high on the tall double doors like the figurehead of a ship, sing the melismatic 'Io ho perduto l'albero', while a group of dancers evoke the waves of the sea with rolling and flowing movements. Three male-female pairs of dancers lean, slide and fall in unison, while maintaining a sense of circularity in their motions that echoes the melisma of the song. The duets finish by leaning foreheads together, before the dancers arch back and break away from each other. Then there is also the Flemish song 'Ick seg adieu', sung by Dockx, which was previously mentioned in Chapter 5. Another example of a secular song is the cantigo 'Ondas do mar', played by Ensemble Micrologus, initially on the Morish guitar, then with the harp, fiddle and flute. Bovi sings to the stormy sea, asking if it has seen her lover and praying to God that he may come home soon. Towards the end of *Myth*, Iris Bouche sings a Vietnamese lullaby, while approaching a seemingly lifeless Alexandra Gilbert on her knees holding a needle and thread. As she advances, she leaves behind her a trace of very long, black trouser legs. She stitches Gilbert's costume on her chest. Meanwhile, Louise, seated on top of the bookshelf, begins to play the sitar and sing 'Bolo bolo'. This traditional Indian song is layered with the Japanese song 'Pilica', sung by Satoshi Kudo. A written fragment of Dante Alighieri's *Divine Comedy* is briefly projected, invoking further medieval Christian ways of thinking; however, due to the Islamic influence on Dante's conceptions of the afterlife, a further iteration of Cherkaoui's transreligious attitude becomes possible to imagine. Likewise, the juxtaposition of the Christian medieval and traditional music with secular songs and those pertaining to other cultures and beliefs serves to highlight the transcultural and transreligious connections between people.

On his fascination with mythology, Cherkaoui explains that he likes that 'it doesn't have a real morality. It is more like cause and effect: "if you do this, then this happens". They are totally untrue stories— I mean, nobody believes them—but at the same time they create an image, and this image helps you to understand a psychological condition' (Cherkaoui qtd. in Cools 8). Between the Islamic and Catholic influences on him as a Muslim growing up in Belgium and the Greek and Roman myths studied at school, his outlook on mythology is implicitly transcultural and transreligious, focused on the connections and overlaps between these different world views. For *Myth*, he also began to work with Hindu archetypes and polytheism, as well as Tarot cards.

To further develop the thinking about Cherkaoui's mise-en-scène, earlier described as kaleidoscopic, through an analysis of *Myth*'s aesthetic, the visual fullness onstage is like a rich tapestry with which spectators are invited to engage in a dramaturgical way. Tapestry is an art for which Flanders has been famous since the thirteenth century and constitutes another medieval influence on this work, in addition to the music and Dante's poetry. Another analogy could be the excessive aesthetic of Flemish Gothic architecture, as can be seen in the cathedral of Antwerp, Cherkaoui's hometown. In an interview with Guy Cools at Sadler's Wells, Cherkaoui mentions taking a journalist who thought the piece was 'too much' to see this cathedral, 'to see the sculpture at the entrance, which is really huge and full of apostles and all of that. You can't take it in, it is just too much. And I asked him, "Do you think the artist is doing too much here?" He understood. When you really focus on the cathedral, you can see the story' (Cherkaoui qtd in Cools 21). Indeed, confirmation that this is a deliberate dramaturgical strategy by the choreographer comes from the work's dramaturg: 'It is a conscious choice by

Larbi to be "all-inclusive" and not to reject any of the images proposed by his dancers, to create a multi-layered visual stream of (un)conscious-ness similar to that of dream associations in which it is both impossible to isolate an image or remember the whole' (Cools 88).

Rather than tapestry or gothic architecture, others have likened *Myth* to the late medieval Flemish paintings by Pieter Bruegel the Elder or Hieronymus Bosch (Micrologus). Their paintings are filled with small scenes depicting popular, social acts, such as children's games, or mys-tic or moralistic imagery, such as the deadly sins, depictions of hell, or people acting out known proverbs. A reviewer of a recent exhibition of Bosch's paintings remarks that 'there is always so much to do in [Bosch's painting] The Garden of Earthly Delights' (Jones). In Bruegel's work, the 'fundamentally disconnected manner of portrayal' has been identi-fied as a key characteristic of the peasant characters in his paintings, each acting separate from and oblivious to the others' (Franits 203). The viewer's gaze is drawn into each of these small scenes in succession, in a time-based process that emphasises discovery of the finer detail. In *Myth*, because there is so much simultaneous activity in different areas of the stage space, on top of a time-based barrage of one image following the previous, it is impossible for spectators to take in everything at once. Instead, the spectator's gaze is directed from one small scene to the next; or, at times, the gaze is not directed but free to roam. The realisation that Cherkaoui's mise-en-scène, inspired by a medieval aesthetic, is intent on overwhelming spectators and inviting them into a decentred, time-based process of discovery, further qualifies the kaleidoscope image. The mise-en-scène is not simply about multi-layered, geometric shifts away from the centre; it is packed with confronting images that carry dense meanings and social, moral and or political implications. What follows is only one example from *Myth* to give the reader an impression of the simultaneity, juxtaposition and time-based succession of micro-stories Cherkaoui stages in the work.

Jalet, growling and on all fours like a wolf, disappears under Dockx's skirt. She drops her fan and contracts her upper body, then arches it back. She gasps. Her hands tremble, along with her skirt. In the back-ground, Ulrika Kinn Svensson lies on top of Louise and thrusts her pelvis into Louise's, making love to her shadow and therefore, perhaps, a part of herself. Dockx's screams become louder and louder, until she emits a high-pitched howl. She grabs onto a cross-dressed Darryl E. Woods's waist as he walks past. Bouche pulls Jalet from under Dockx's skirt and drags him away. Likewise, Leboutte pulls Svensson away from Louise, prompting Svensson to project her sexual desire suddenly on Leboutte, who rejects her saying that she does not want it in French. Woods and Dockx have begun to sway from side to side in a slow dance. Simone Sorini sings the song 'Lucente Stella' while a series of sensual male-female duets ensue. The song addresses heartbreak from an unrequited love. Marc Wagemans and Dockx resume their scene of flirtation and rejection with which the work as a whole opened. Now, Dockx, wearing the white wedding dress, is being pleaded with by Wagemans who stands in front of her and reaches both arms out to her and brings his hands to his heart, repeatedly. She keeps fanning her face with her hand in an aloof manner, avoiding eye contact. Damien Fournier and Louise embark on a sensuous and acrobatic duet, in which her contorted body, leg tucked behind her neck, is carried and swung around by him. Bouche and Jalet also dance a duet, until they resume their roles of mistress and growling animal. Woods dances elegantly in front of an upstanding antique mirror. His movements start as balletic poses and transform into body rolls.

Myth is deeply permeated by Jungian psychoanalytical concepts, particularly choreographed representations of the shadow and the circumambulation of symbols in dream analysis, and the psychoanalyst Carl Gustav Jung's writing is cited by one of the performers on stage. Such indicators of the collective unconscious, visible and audible in the staged work, directly informed the construction of the analytical methodology employed in this chapter. Cherkaoui's choreographic rendition of these Jungian concepts demands an exploration of their implications for dramaturgical analysis and understandings of meaning-making processes. A review in the *Los Angeles Times* likens the work itself to a dream: 'Like one of those dreams that are simultaneously frightening and alluring, Sidi Larbi Cherkaoui's "Myth" [...] trades in things that don't quite add up [...]. Dreams are dense with meaning yet don't make sense, after all, and as Cherkaoui proposes, neither do humankind's cherished myths' (Wolf).

Cools, who worked with Cherkaoui on *Myth* as dramaturg, and Lou Cope, who observed the creation process as part of her research, both reveal the change in the work's focus throughout its process. The starting point for the work was the idea of trauma. '[Cherkaoui] is interested in exploring the ways people carry past trauma with them, in their minds or in their bodies' (Cope). For Cools, the central question of the work was 'How can a certain event mark an individual forever?' 'To avoid this directness [of simply focusing on trauma], the choreographer tempers his approach by saying: yes, but trauma is related in German to *Traum* and *Traum* also means dream' (Cools 83).

In his writing on dream analysis, Jung (*Dream Analysis*) articulates a number of affinities between dreams and theatre. He likens the structure of individual dreams to that of Greek drama and considers the occurrence of theatrical settings in dreams 'an anticipation of the process of analysis' (Jung *Dream Analysis* 13). Jung foregrounds the theatrical in his writing on dreams, stating that 'a dream is a theatre in which the dreamer is himself the scene, the player, the prompter, the producer, the author, the public, and the critic' (*Structure and Dynamics* 266). Cherkaoui's original impulse for creating *Myth* was to examine how people deal with trauma and how they can heal themselves (Cope). The therapeutic potential of the work becomes apparent in its dream-like imagery which coerces the spectators into a confrontation with aspects of the Self that they may have repressed. Cherkaoui likens this to the workings of homeopathy, 'where the active ingredient is always diluted in other stuff. It's not just pure vitamins, which are sometimes too harsh, too radical, too clean. Sometimes you need it coming from an apple. The body is very smart; it can take things. And I believe the audience is also very smart and can take out what it needs for itself' (Cherkaoui qtd. in Cools 19).

Meaning is by no means evident and straightforward in *Myth*. Dance sequences, songs, instrumental music, monologues and nonsensical conversations in a variety of languages are layered on top of each other in a complex dramaturgy, set in an overcrowded space, and the spectators are ultimately left to their own devices to 'make sense' of this barrage of theatrical images. Another way of describing *Myth* is that it is 'multi-focused, multi-layered and consequently consciously denies the notion of one fixed truth in favour of multiple equally (in)valid truths that are crucially open to multiple interpretation' (Cope). The composition process is described as 'a collective assemblage' in which none of the performers, nor Cherkaoui, knew how the different ingredients of the work would end up fitting together (Cope). In this, Cherkaoui deliberately sought out complexity and multiplicity. Cherkaoui says: 'As we were making material a lot of things got created and all of them made sense to the people involved. Then what most directors do is "kill your darlings"; you have to cut, cut, cut, cut... [..] and I thought, "what if I don't; what if I keep everything, what if everything gets a place, what if I don't reject anything?" [...] I wanted everything to get a space [...] like in an encyclopaedia' (Cherkaoui qtd. in Cools 19). Cope emphasises that none of the makers of *Myth* are in control of its signification: 'It is a third thing that exceeds the knowledge of all those that made it. And just as Cherkaoui has made his own sense out of nonsense, both we the audience, and they the performers, are left to make our own sense of what is being presented and experienced' (Cope). For the performers, 'this search for meaning will continue throughout the tour', whereas for a spectator-researcher like me, who is professionally invested in working to understand the dramaturgical implications of the work, it encourages multiple viewings and a revisiting of the work's imagery time and time again (Cope).

The following sections will analyse the implications of Cherkaoui's choreographing of Jungian concepts, namely shadows and circumambulation, which Jung suggests is an important approach in dream analysis. The final section of this chapter will investigate how Cherkaoui circumambulates the religious symbol of the cross and therefore invites the spectator to engage in a personal circumambulation of different elements of the work as a strategy to recover meaning from the theatrical imagery. By exploring Jung's writings on excavation and circumambulation in dream analysis, possible parallels with his concepts are extended to the continuous macro dramaturgy of the spectator. I argue that dream analysis, and by extension also Jungian analysis in general, strongly corresponds to dramaturgical practice.

SHADOWS

The set, collaboratively designed by Cherkaoui and Wim Van de Cappelle, is characterised by tall double doors in the back wall which dominate the stage. Next to the doors are a bookshelf with leather-bound books, human and animal skulls, a skeleton sitting on a chair, and an antique mirror. When the audience enters the auditorium, six protagonists, clothed in a variety of colours and styles, are already in this space—a waiting room? A library? Purgatory? The idea of purgatory is given support at the start of *Myth*'s second chapter, when a quote from Dante's *Divine Comedy*, an allegorical poem from the fourteenth century, is projected onto the back wall. The text describes the author's journey through the afterlife, each part dealing with hell, purgatory and heaven respectively. With regard to purgatory, Dante imagines this to exist as a place on earth in the southern hemisphere that is governed by time passing, as he can see the sun moving. His use of the word 'ombra' carries a double meaning: it refers to both the shadow cast by the body and the transformation of the soul in the afterlife into a shade, a virtual being that is impressed onto the space surrounding the body and takes on bodily functions of its own. As previously introduced, the passage through purgatory is for souls who must go through a time-bound process of purification before their earthly sins are forgiven and they can enter heaven. While at first glance, Dante's conception of the afterlife strongly represents a medieval Christian way of thinking, scholars have argued there is a substantial Islamic influence in his *Divine Comedy* (Ziolkowski). In the light of Cherkaoui's transreligious outlook, he may have been interested in this relationship between Christianity and Islam (Fig. 6.1).

At the start of the work, most of the protagonists, Leboutte, Svensson, Dockx, Wagemans and Woods, sit quietly on benches and chairs, while a nerdy-looking boy with glasses, Milan Herich, flicks through some books. Suddenly, eight dancers crawl on the floor, entering the stage space through gates, nooks or crannies in the walls. Dressed completely in black, they align their bodies with those of the protagonists that were already present. The performers in black adopt body positions that are identical to those of the protagonists, but lying on the floor, in the horizontal rather than vertical plane, as if they are embodying the protagonists' shadows cast on the ground by the light. The shadows start whispering and moving nervously around the protagonists, stalking them and manipulating them into certain actions. Someone sneezes. People stand up and walk around to stretch their legs. Woods trips over one of his shadows. Across the stage, a few other protagonists are now being followed by shadows on the floor, who imitate their movements. These shadows can be interpreted as embodied representations of the Jungian notion of the shadow:

> The thing you have buried grows fat while you grow thin. If you get rid of qualities you don't like by denying them, you become more and more unaware of what you are, you declare yourself more and more non-exist-ent, and your devils will grow fatter and fatter. (Jung *Dream Analysis* 53)

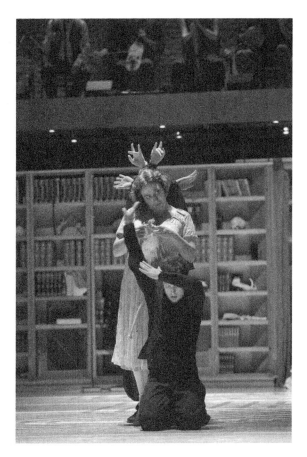

Fig. 6.1 Christine Leboutte and Milan Herich in *Myth* (Photo by Laurent Philippe)

The protagonists are physically confronted with the dark, animalistic sides of their personality, which are now inescapable as they incessantly invade the protagonists' personal space two or three at a time. Svensson dances a playful duet with her shadow, embodied by Peter Jaško, whose presence she seems to have suddenly become aware of. She tries to catch the shadow with her hands as if it were a tangible person, unsuccessfully, as he constantly slips through her fingers. This can be seen as a choreographing of the Jungian concept of individuation, the process of self-realisation by which a person integrates the conscious ego with both the individual and the collective unconscious into the total Self. The term 'Self' is capitalised by Jung because it 'transcends the ego and inheres the age-old capacities of the species' (Stevens 45). Individuation entails a confrontation with one's unconscious shadow; its expressions are examined in order for the individual to come to terms with it. Svensson's shadow is teasing her, mocking her attempts to literally come to grips with those repressed qualities of the Self. Her movements become confused and dizzy, as she is now surrounded by a multiplicity of shadows: three dancers as well as the multiple natural shadows on the floor caused by the theatre lights.

If Svensson was aware of her shadows and at least attempting to control them, Woods is far less empowered in his process of becoming aware of his shadows. Cross-dressed in high heels, a blue satin pantsuit and fringed bob wig, he becomes the victim in a haunted scene, in which his shadows frighten him by pushing random books off the shelf, placing an animal skull on the chair on which he is about to sit, and tickling him with their hair and the hand of a skeleton. Woods reacts by squealing first, then laughing to himself in disbelief, as if he is just imagining the haunting, but then his screams become louder and quicker in succession, until he shouts at himself to snap out of it. The piercing sound of the bagpipes ensues, along with a rhythmical percussion pattern, to which Svensson and the shadow chorus dance in unison. They walk forwards and backwards, lift their knees, fold in their arms, drop to the ground and roll repeatedly. Meanwhile, Leboutte runs around the stage and fervently knocks on the double doors, seeking to be let out of this haunted place. The scene builds to a climax, with more instruments joining in, including the natural trumpet and castanets. Svensson convulses as if she is possessed, abruptly turning in her legs and her arm in angular shapes and dropping to her knees and eventually lifelessly onto her side.

Three shadows, Kudo, Fournier and Jalet move on all fours and growl, evoking the image of wolves. Fournier grabs onto bandages around Leboutte's wrists with his teeth and drags her towards Svensson's body. It occurs to me that Leboutte's character might have attempted to commit suicide and that might be why she is wearing those bandages. This image fits with the notion of *Myth* evoking a waiting room filled with sinners waiting in purgatory. To instrumental bagpipe and percussive music, the three wolf-like figures pull Svensson's limbs with their teeth and revive her, carrying her around like a queen. She now looks powerful and sexy, and the wolves appear to worship her like a queen. She flicks wolf Kudo's long locks. Her attempt to come to grips with her shadows has failed and is abandoned. Completely manipulated by the embodied shadows into these movements, she can be considered to exemplify the cardinal sins of pride and lust, drawing upon elements of Christian morality. The three wolves tumble over each other's backs in a motion resembling an infinity symbol. They form a tower by jumping onto each other's hips while crouching. They form a cluster, in which the three bodies advance downstage as one like the mythical three-headed dog Cerberus, who guards the underworld, suggesting a link with the afterlife.

Svensson calls Jalet to come to her, but he growls, then bites her arm and her leg. She shakes him off every time and they begin a well-matched fight. Svensson then roars loudly in a very deep voice. The penetrating sound of the bagpipes is layered over her roars. Kudo approaches her, holding a black martial arts staff in front of his body, making very small circles with it. Svensson stamps her heels and smashes the staff with her book. Kudo blocks her blows and offers resistance when she tries to push him over. Goffredo Degli Esposti, on the bagpipes, matches their dynamics responsively, emphasising every blow with an accent in the music. After Kudo has put the staff down, Svensson tries to catch him, but he evades her grip every time. She is totally exasperated and Kudo stands behind her, holds her arm and strokes her hair, gently singing the 'Edo' lullaby.

Svensson walks away, as Bouche joins Kudo in a duet in which they face each other and, with their wrists connected, they make circular arm movements, while both singing the lullaby. Herich then suddenly pierces the staff between Kudo's arm and side, as if impaling him. He shakes Kudo's body off the staff. Kudo, however, is instantly revived, leading Herich to continue his attacks. Fournier enters and pushes Herich away, seemingly to care for Kudo. However, Fournier and Kudo in turn enter into an endless cycle of attacking, 'dying' and being revived. Several other dancers join in with the fight. Meanwhile, Bouche, Gilbert and Jalet perform a movement sequence in the corners of the stage space in which they fall to their knees and bounce up and down. They spin and arch back, repeatedly falling to their knees.

Cherkaoui's stated starting point for *Myth*, namely the ways in which individuals carry their past traumas with them, seems significant with regard to the exchanges between the protagonists and other dancers dressed in black resembling their shadows. The power play within the manifold interactions between six protagonists and their shadows visualises the psychoanalytical notion that people's actions may be driven by aspects of their personality that they are trying to repress, as they drift into consciousness. In this first section, analysis of the dramaturgical elements indicates that the protagonists' experience of being confronted by their Jungian shadows may in fact serve as the process of purification that Christian morality defines as purgatory, which can be seen to correspond to the Jungian process of individuation.

Away from this dominant Christian perspective on the work, influences from Eastern thought were also at work on Cherkaoui and Cools during the creation process, which have equally shaped the choreographic approach to the notion of shadows in the work. Approaching human duality as 'complementary, coexisting and even cooperating entities—as perfectly symbolized by the Chinese yin and yang alternation', the work as a whole is organised around 'the notion of somatic and energetic opposites [as a] binding theme: how to integrate the shadow side, the animal in us' (Cools 87–89). To this end, Cherkaoui actively exposes contradictory behaviour within the characters. For example, Leboutte is a character who takes care of the subordinated Wagemans, while she denies and rejects O'Hara as her own son. In one scene, she sits on a chair and closes her legs, but is squirming. A hand is pushing up from underneath her skirt and she tries to push it back down with both hands. She pants. She kneels and two arms reach out from underneath her skirt. She shakes her head and tries to push the arms back, as if she is giving birth to an unwanted child whom she is trying to push back into the womb. O'Hara's head and naked torso emerge. He reaches up to Leboutte's breasts, but she cries and shouts no. When he is fully 'born', wearing nothing but beige underpants, Leboutte tries to walk away, but he grabs on to her leg. She pivots and swings her other leg over his head. He jumps on her back, swings round and slides down her chest, as if trying to find his mother's nipple. She continually pushes him away. Coming out stronger in this struggle, Leboutte kicks O'Hara off and onto the ground, and runs over to knock on the double doors, quietly calling out for her own mother. Cherkaoui is interested in this multiplicity and complexity within a person, akin to Eastern theatre forms, in which 'the actor incarnates more than one character, both good and evil, man and woman. The actor is everything, everybody. One is capable of changing perspective all the time' (Cherkaoui qtd. in Cools 89). *Myth* opens up the thinking around how people's actions are influenced by the traumas of their past. The Christian medieval notions of sin and purgatory are recast through the Jungian shadow to emphasise the process of individuation. The tensions within the complex, contradictory behaviours of some of the characters shine yet another light on individuals' motivations, through the Eastern notion of yin and yang alternation. These are some of the readings of *Myth*, achieved through repeated viewings, impressions of the creative process gleaned from observation and the accounts by Cope and Cools, and an excavation of elements readily visible in the work. These choreographic elements include the link between Jung through the reciting of one of his texts, which will be explored in more detail in the next section, the projected quotes by Dante, the choreographed shadow figures and their power play with the protagonists. The next section will delve further into the Christian iconography of the cross Cherkaoui evokes through his choreography.

CIRCUMAMBULATING THE DYNAMIC CROSS

This section will explore the potential of Jungian excavation of dreams with reference to a significant scene from *Myth*, in terms of its religious implications. Before engaging in this detailed analysis, however, it is useful to consider another connection between the unconscious and theatre in relation to *Myth*. In 'The Unconscious as Mise-en-Scène', the philosopher Jean-François Lyotard established a parallel between Freudian dreamwork and the mise-en-scène of nineteenth-century opera, arguing that all primary messages of the unconscious must be staged in order for people to access them. The staging of the unconscious involves a number of complex operations, referred to as dreamwork. Dramaturgy, like mise-en-scène, can for our purposes also be considered a kind of dreamwork, especially because Cherkaoui often complicates his theatrical images so that they are beyond simple signification. Dramaturgy requires a creative and open-minded approach, similarly to Jung's approach of 'creative work with symbols' (Stevens 87).

It is the ways in which spectators might approach Cherkaoui's works that benefit from the analogy with Jungian therapeutic methods. In this analogy, Jung's concept of 'circumambulation' becomes especially useful. Jung first encountered this concept in his exploration of Eastern *mandala* symbolism and ritual, and later applied the term to his concepts of individuation and the Self (Coward 51). His emphasis on 'walking around' refers to the Latin roots of the word, and it is in this capacity that the term becomes productive when applied to the theatrical images in Cherkaoui's dramaturgy. For Jung, dream analysis involves circumambulating the symbols in the dream so that they may 'reveal their different facets to consciousness' (Stevens 87). It bears resemblance to archaeology:

> As he [Jung] often said, he approached a dream as if it were an undeciphered text and he used all his archaeological instincts in the endeavour. Only when one has excavated the personal, cultural, and archetypal foundations of the dream is one in a position to appreciate its implications. Then, as one strolls round the site of one's excavations the dream's architecture stands revealed, together with a sense of what the architect was seeking to achieve, and where all his creative energy could lead. It is a delicate process of sifting, cataloguing, and comparing, requiring much imaginative flair: the dream must never be excavated to destruction, but its atmosphere savoured and its message left intact. (Stevens 94)

By circumambulating the theatrical images of *Myth* and unravelling the dramaturgical dreamwork at play, spectators may begin to demythologise some of the work's more obscure dramaturgic content.

Halfway through the performance, Svensson recites Jung's text 'The Christ Within' (Jung 280), proclaiming how Christ is within each person, equating the figure of Christ to the potential of the Self within each human being waiting to be realised.

'From my observations, I found that the modern unconscious has a tendency to produce a psychological condition which we find, for instance, in medieval mysticism. You find certain things in Meister Eckhart; you find many things in Gnosticism. You find the idea of the Adam Kadmon in every man—the Christ within. Christ is the second Adam, which is also, in exotic religions, the idea of the Atman or the complete man, the original man, the "all-round" man by Plato, symbolised by a circle or a drawing with circular motifs. You find all these things in medieval mysticism; in alchemical literature, in the New Testament, of course, in Paul. But it is an absolutely consistent development of the idea of the Christ within; and the argument is that it is absolutely immoral to allow Christ to suffer for us, that he has suffered enough, that we should carry our own sins for once and not shift them off onto Christ—that we should carry them all. Christ expresses the same idea when he says, "I appear in the least of your brethren"; and what about it... If the least of your brethren should be yourself, what about it then? Then you get the intimation that Christ is not to be the least in your life, that we have a brother in ourselves who is really the least of our brethren, much worse than the poor beggar whom you feed. That is, in ourselves we have a shadow; we have a very bad fellow in ourselves, a very poor man, and he has to be accepted. What has Christ done—let us be quite banal about it—what has Christ done when we consider him as an entirely human creature? Christ was disobedient to his mother; Christ was disobedient to his tradition; he carried through his hypothesis to the bitter end. How was Christ born? In the greatest misery. Who was his father? He was an illegitimate child—humanly the most miserable situation: a poor girl having a little son. That is our symbol, that is ourselves; we are all that. This is modern psychology. This is the future. This is the true future. This is the future of which I know but, of course, the historical future might be quite different. But I do not care for a historic future at all; I am not concerned with it. I am only concerned with the fulfilment of that will that is in every individual. My history is only the history of those individuals who are going to fulfil their hypotheses. That is the whole problem. That is my standpoint. That is the problem. That is my standpoint'.

In this text recited by Svensson in *Myth*, Jung traces a number of transcultural connections within the figure of Christ. He is inviting his readers to conceive of Christ as an archetype and a transcultural and transreligious figure. This may be the reason why Svensson and Cherkaoui have opted to include this particular excerpt in isolation.

For all her pontificating using Jung's words, Svensson still seems to be struggling with a few issues of her own. As has been introduced in Chapter 5, in the context of language confusion and non-translation, she quotes the text in a pedantic voice, lecturing to Wagemans, a performer with Down's syndrome, who has knelt down to kiss her hand. The text is written in the first person, so Svensson brings Jung's voice directly into the theatre. While she singles out Wagemans to 'be taught' this complex idea, she subordinates him physically. Wagemans moves across the stage on hands and knees, a leash around his neck held by Svensson. Svensson puts her foot on Wagemans's back, her crossed forearms resting on her knee, as she puts on her glasses. At one point, she militantly stands on Wagemans's back, exclaiming the key points of Jung's speech in a droning voice. The whole scene is drowned out by the performance of the song 'Brumas e mors' by Ensemble Micrologus and the other performers, so that the Jung text becomes very hard to hear and follow. This is an act, by Cherkaoui, of simultaneously introducing the idea of Jungian psychoanalytical writing and undermining it with a song from the oral tradition. Nevertheless, with this scene, Svensson does, in an indirect way, allude to the arrival of Christ, which comes slightly later on in the work.

Towards the end of *Myth*, it would seem that finally salvation arrives. There is a knock on the tall double doors, from the outside this time. Woods, donning a pearl-coloured evening dress and tiara, and fanning himself, is sitting on the chair next to the doors and asks: 'Who is it?' This is quite funny, as throughout the work, there has been a strong pull of desire from various performers to escape purgatory through these doors. For example, earlier in the work, after the scene in which O'Hara was born, he walks to the doors, which are guarded by five growling men in black. Jalet and Fournier drag O'Hara by the elbows away from the door. O'Hara walks back to the door and is thrown onto the floor by Kudo. O'Hara jumps towards the door, but is caught on the shoulder by Jalet, carried away and placed down. This pattern continues several times, until the three men loudly bark at O'Hara. Given the pull of the big door, it seems unlikely that the protagonists' opening of the doors would be contingent on who is on the other side knocking. Svensson recoils from the door, unsure what will happen next. Fournier, dressed in blue jeans with naked torso, opens the tall double doors and enters through them, his bulky shoulder muscles flexed and his head hanging forward. I am reminded that several years ago when we talked about *Myth*, Cherkaoui likened Fournier's physicality and movement preferences to the image of Atlas, a mythological figure, a Titan who was condemned to hold up the sky for eternity and is often depicted carrying the celestial spheres on his shoulders. The figure of Atlas itself is very rich from a transcultural perspective, in that this Ancient Greek notion was likely influenced by Berber culture and in turn later influenced Greco-Buddhist and Arabian culture and mythology.

Accompanied by the harp and Mauro Borgioni's tenor voice in the song 'Io son un pellegrin', Fournier limps in, using two wooden poles as crutches. He leans one of the poles against his shoulder and spins the other one around to a horizontal position and places it on the back of his neck, while resting both wrists on it. Instantaneously the image of Christ on the cross is evoked. However, Fournier drops to his knees immediately, and hence the Latin cross is inverted, alluding to Saint Peter, who was crucified upside down. Clutching the pole under his chin to control it, he tips it so that it rests on his back; the bottom of the earlier cross has become the top of another, which he now bears on his back like Christ is depicted as doing in the Stations of the Cross, commemorated on Good Friday. He gets back on his feet and spins around, exposing the image of the cross as a dynamic and three-dimensional object. Borgioni sings the lilting *melismata* of the Florentine song, which translates as: 'A pilgrim am I, that alms do seek. For God's mercy, chanting. Singing go I with tuneful voice. A fair countenance and a golden braid. Naught have I but staff and purse, and sing, and sing, but no one answers. And when I think of going to the second step, a contrary wind comes storming' (Micrologus). As in earlier iterations of *melismatic* singing, the long succession of notes, travelling up and down the scale and embellishing relatively simple lyrics, seem to open up the space in the melody, inviting the listener to indulge in it and let its meaning sink in on an affective level. So, too, does the theatrical image invite the spectator to linger with it.

The two poles, crossed diagonally behind Fournier's neck, have become crutches again. This X-shaped cross invokes the cross on which Saint Andrew was crucified. Fournier's manipulation of the cross as a fluid symbol thus evokes imagery of Christ and his apostles at one fell swoop. He rotates underneath the poles and edges back until they come apart, at which moment he moves to thrust the poles into his torso like spears. After a brief moment during which his arms and torso hang drooped down over the poles, he moves to pull them away, letting his body exaggerate the reaction of the tugging. He leaps forward into a wide stance, so that his feet are connected to the bottom of the two poles, now resting vertically on the floor on either side of his body. Fournier swings from left to right, as if external forces are pulling him into opposite directions. He spins one of the poles and places it down, reaching across his body to the other side, then repeats the same action with the other pole. He rests one pole on his shoulder vertically and slowly sweeps it around, as if he is taking aim with a bow and arrow. Having shot the arrow, it immediately turns around and hits him in the stomach, invoking the death of another Christian martyr, Saint Sebastian. He then falls to the ground and holds the poles in an inverted Latin cross shape again, only to rise back to his feet and the horizontal pole with it, until a conventional Latin cross is shown. He places the two poles on either side of his body again and hooks his right leg around one of the poles. He moves forward, using the poles as crutches, as if his leg was amputated. He spins both poles counterclockwise, but gently twists his upper body, so that the spinning poles trace a sideways figure of eight, resembling an infinity symbol. This symbol, wrapped around the bars of a Latin cross, forms part of the cross of Saint Boniface, an Anglo-Saxon Christian missionary. However, it is also considered a variant of the *ouroboros*, an Ancient Egyptian image of a snake eating its own head, symbolising the cyclical nature of life and death, but also introspection. Considering the connections to Indian thought and the concept of Kundalini, or the coiled serpent, this evocation of the infinity symbol—a key choreographic images that shapes much of Cherkaoui's circular, never-ending movement sequences—again in a dynamic form, invites the spectator to take into account the transcultural connections that have shaped it (Fig. 6.2).

The other performers gather around Fournier expectantly and watch him freeing himself from the poles by pushing them away from him one by one. As soon as he gets to his feet, they advance towards him and clutch on to him and each other in a tight embrace. Step by step, Fournier pushes this huddle of people towards the double doors. Ensemble Micrologus sings the *a capella* song 'Sepulto Domino', about the tomb of Christ and His resurrection. The group hug disperses and the performers kneel, while Fournier lifts and carries each performer one by one, paying brief individual attention to each. He lifts Jalet high up in the air and gently places him down again. He assists Gilbert in performing a slow and controlled cartwheel, holding her waist. O'Hara and Jaško grab on to his ankle while he walks forward, and Louise comes tumbling down over his back and shoulders. He drapes Leboutte over his back and carries her across to the other side, before gently placing her down. Herich leaps towards him and he catches him in his arms, spinning. The brief moment of contact with Fournier seems to have a healing effect on them, as they emerge from it calm and cleansed. It is as if he has washed away their sin. Then, they clutch on to him all together again, resembling the fullness and tragic display of bodies of the baroque paintings of Peter Paul Rubens, another Antwerp resident. Fournier pulls away from them again, but keeps attracting their bodies like a magnet. More embraces follow, now two at a time briefly being held by Fournier and placed down. Yet again the mass of people gets up and he slightly recoils. Their hands grab on to his naked torso. Finally, he pushes the

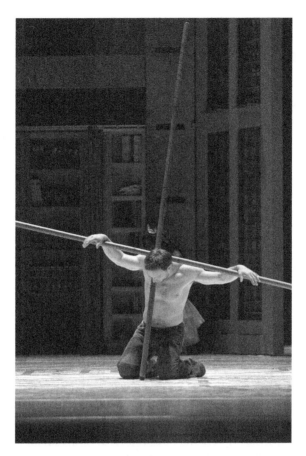

Fig. 6.2   Damien Fournier in *Myth* (Photo by Laurent Philippe)

huddle back towards and through the double doors. Still looking down, he closes the doors once they are all through. I notice that Woods is still sitting on the chair; he had no part in this scene of salvation. His time in purgatory is not yet finished. In a final image, Bouche, who was standing in front of Fournier, drops down and drags herself away from him, tracing his growing shadow with her long, black trouser legs diagonally across the stage.

This final scene in *Myth* seems to suggest a way of analysing the dense theatrical images in the work as a whole. Fournier seems to play with the idea of 'becoming Christ', spinning and balancing his two poles and forming different cross shapes with them. Fournier bears the cross on his back. He hangs on the cross. He transforms the cross into weapons, spears and a bow and arrow. There is never a nail securing the two poles into one fixed shape: the fluid, flexible cross only becomes itself through movements performed by Fournier. It vanishes as soon as it appears, so he can never be put on this cross. The reference to the crucifix alludes to one of the most prevalent myths of Christianity: that of self-sacrifice. Christ underwent torture and died for the sins of the people, so that they could become closer to God. It is believed there is redemption through suffering. The music in this scene, 'Io son un pellegrin', refers to pilgrimage, another form of self-sacrifice, which for Christians in past centuries involved undertaking long, sometimes dangerous, journeys to the location of Christ's death and resurrection. It is believed that some pilgrims also travelled around for the sake of wandering without a specific destination, for ascetic reasons. If Fournier is considered a pilgrim, an eternal wanderer, this is reflected in the way the cross is presented in this scene: the image wanders in front of the spectators' eyes and is constantly transformed. At one moment, he lies on the ground underneath an inverted Latin cross; besides being associated with Satanism and therefore considered disrespectful, this cross symbol is also believed to be a Catholic symbol of humility and unworthiness, following the legend that Saint Peter asked to be crucified upside down.

In this scene, Cherkaoui plays with possibilities for signification beyond the obvious: with each image of the cross that Fournier creates through movement, the dream image of the cross is shifted further. In effect, what Cherkaoui demonstrates is a form of dream analysis at work, circumambulating this symbol so that its different inherent tacit layers become apparent (Jung). The flexible cross that Cherkaoui offers in this scene equally eludes dogmatic signification. Through the scene, the other characters gaze at Fournier in amazement; they seem to force him into the role of being their saviour. At the end of the scene, they literally cling on to him in a tight group embrace. Almost suffocating, Fournier slowly pushes the group of people towards and then through the open doors in the back wall. He closes the door and stays in the waiting space with his shadow growing, personified by Bouche. This growing shadow created by Bouche's trouser legs perhaps indicates that he is human and mortal after all. There is no resurrection. Fournier, like everyone else, is left with his shadow side to deal with in the process of individuation.

Returning to the idea of dreamwork, when we try to recall and recount a dream, the formerly vivid landscape of the dream becomes distant, while we work towards a conceivable structure of the dream and attempt to solidify it. Narrating a dream, 'we focus on detail and then move on to the next in order to make sense of the total content. Dream-content, however, is more like a sculpture than a film. In a dream, the whole is given all at once and is encoded in the image' (Sonenberg 31). This apt description also applies Cherkaoui's theatrical images in *Myth*: they have the same sculptural qualities, encapsulating many fragments of ideas in a non-linear, and simultaneous dramaturgy. They may therefore leave the spectator feeling incapable of recounting the performance they have just witnessed, just as it is impossible to relive and retell a dream. An engaged spectatorship that includes an excavation of the multi-layered iconography in the choreography is a viable strategy to grapple with the complexity of the work's dramaturgy and bridge the gap between affect and consciousness. In this final scene where Fournier plays with the shifting images of the cross, Cherkaoui demonstrates circumambulation as a kind of dream analysis at work, unpicking the different layers encapsulated within a single symbol. As a result, *Myth* is more than just the equivalent of a dream, or a staging of the unconscious: it also operates on a dream-analytical level in recovering meaning from these symbols. Jung refuses a dogmatic approach and the idea of a fixed meaning of symbols; similarly, Cherkaoui's choreography eludes singular and final signification.

Jung's psychoanalytical theory deeply permeates the dramaturgical layers of *Myth*. There are similarities to the Freudian complex staging of the unconscious, as Cherkaoui equally complicates his dramaturgy, playing with disguise, distortions and latent dream content. The spectators are invited to employ their active imaginations to engage with the complex, multi-layered dramaturgy; the work invites an archaeological analytical approach very similar to Jungian dream analysis. The analogy of dreams and dramaturgy reflects some specific ideas about the political functions of theatre performance. As demonstrated in the example of the cross scene, Cherkaoui uses fluid, flexible and ambiguous images which estrange the audience. These images are dream-like because they are inaccessible and obscure, which may encourage the audience to examine them in a new light. An affective engagement with the work alone may be a powerful experience for the spectator. However, Cherkaoui also offers the audience a way into the therapeutic process of dream analysis, leaving the spectators with questions about their own position, and their own attitudes. That way, they learn more about themselves as spectators, and by extension about society in general—in Jungian terms, they can be therefore seen to begin to engage in a process of individuation. Performers frequently bring in foreign languages and 'Other' cultural elements to the staged works. Watching these works, spectators have to trust their associations. The dramaturgies no longer privilege a single, unified (Western) knowledge base and cannot be read without the spectator's active and engaged spectatorship.

In *Myth*, religion is explored and evaluated by Cherkaoui as another kind of myth. Due to the large amount of references in the work to Jungian psychoanalysis (the archetype of the shadow, the reciting of the Jungian text 'The Christ Within'), the previous section developed an analytical tool for spectators based on Jungian dream analysis with which to engage with the various latent layers that are enveloped in this work. The scene in which the cross is choreographed as a fluid and shifting symbol is poignant in this regard. It shows a kind of circumambulation at work; the symbol of the cross itself wanders in front of the eye of the spectator without ever being fixed, inviting the spectator to recover meanings from it through dreamwork, and challenging reductive interpretation and singular meaning. By presenting religion as myth, Cherkaoui can be seen to choreograph against religious fundamentalism in a way that is different from the one discussed in Chapter 4 in relation to *Apocrifu* (2007). The earlier discussion of Cherkaoui's choreographing the intertextuality of religious texts, guarding against the violence and volatility potentially resulting from literal interpretations of religious texts, is stretched further by the visual, choreographic circumambulation of the cross. Both choreographic strategies invite spectators to question received meanings and regard them as unfixed and fluid. More broadly and methodologically, Cherkaoui invites the spectator to engage creatively with the images and texts with which his works are infused, in a way that is macro-dramaturgical and ongoing.

Circumambulation, the continuous resignification of objects and dancing bodies through a choreographic play of continuous repurposing, occurs in several of Cherkaoui's works. This spectatorial strategy becomes relevant in the signification process too, as a parallel was established between the 'walking around' symbols when excavating dreams during analysis and the dramaturgical labour on the part of the spectator, who engages with the performance both in-the-moment and retrospectively. In many ways, this manipulation of objects returns in the works for which Cherkaoui collaborated with visual artist Antony Gormley: *zero degrees* (co-choreographed with Akram Khan, 2005), *Sutra* (2008) and *Babel^(words)* (co-choreographed with Jalet, 2010). In *zero degrees*, the latex dummies, casts of Khan's and Cherkaoui's bodies, are treated as witnesses, allies, enemies and dead bodies. In *Sutra*, a set of 21 life-size wooden boxes are designed with proportions that allow their manifold rearrangement and rebuilding. Manipulated by the monks of the Shaolin Temple, they are transformed into a multitude of meanings: pillars, a maze, coffins, bunk beds, a boat, skyscrapers, a lotus flower opening, dominoes. Chapter 3 analysed these works in more detail. Furthermore, as will be discussed in further detail next in Chapter 7, the aluminium frames in *Babel^(words)* similarly wander in front of the eye of the spectator, demonstrating how space and territory are continuously manipulated by architecture. His wider application of the choreographic strategy of circumambulation indicates that it is effective beyond the particular context of religion as myth. However, circumambulation as a choreographic strategy does not rely on the manipulation of objects alone; it also applies to the dancing body in its own right and to the relationships between dancers. For example, in *Rien de Rien* (2000), analysed in Chapter 2, Cherkaoui performs a lengthy sequence of hand gestures by continuously manipulating one hand with the other into a peace sign, a military salute, a Hitler salute, and so on. He shows that, by carrying out very small adjustments with one hand to the other, subtle and drastic shifts in meanings occur.

Bibliography

Cools, Guy. *Body: Language #1. The Mythic Body: Guy Cools with Sidi Larbi Cherkaoui*. London: Sadler's Wells. 2012. Print.

———. *In-Between Dance Cultures: On the Migratory Artistic Identity of Sidi Larbi Cherkaoui and Akram Khan*. Antennae Series. Amsterdam: Valiz, 2015. Print.

Cope, Lou. 'Sidi Larbi Cherkaoui: Myth (2007)—Mapping the Multiple'. *Making Contemporary Theatre: International Rehearsal Processes*. Ed. Harvie, Jen & Lavender, Andy. Manchester: Manchester University Press, 2010. 39–58. Print.

Coward, Harold. *Jung and Eastern Thought*. Albany: State University of New York Press, 1995. Print.

Franits, Wayne. *Dutch Seventeenth-Century Genre Painting*. New Haven, CT: Yale University Press. 2004. Print.

Jones, Jonathan. 'Hieronymus Bosch Review—A Heavenly Host of Delights on the Way to Hell'. *The Guardian*. 2016. Web. Accessed: 30 August 2017. <https://www.theguardian.com/artanddesign/2016/feb/11/hieronymus-bosch-review-a-heavenly-host-of-delights-on-the-road-to-hell>.

Jung, Carl Gustav. (trans. by R.F.C. Hull). *The Structure and Dynamics of the Psyche*. London: Routledge and Kegan Paul, 1960. Print.

———. (ed. Aniela Jaffé; trans. Richard and Clara Winston) *Memories, Dreams, Reflections*. London and Glasgow: Random House, 1963. Print.

———. (trans. R.F.C. Hull) *The Symbolic Life: Miscellaneous Writings*. London: Routledge and Kegan Paul, 1977. Print.

———. (ed. William McGuire) *Dream Analysis: Notes of the Seminar Given in 1928–1930*. London: Routledge & Kegan Paul, 1984. Print.

Lyotard, Jean-François. 'The Unconscious as Mise-en-Scène'. *Mimesis, Masochism, & Mime: The Politics of Theatricality in Contemporary French Thought*. Ed. Murray, Tim. Ann Arbor: University of Michigan Press, 1997. 163–174. Print.

Micrologus. *Myth—Sidi Larbi Cherkaoui: The Music*. 2007. Booklet with CD.

Sonenberg, Janet. *Dreamwork for Actors*. London: Routledge, 2003. Print.

Stevens, Anthony. *Jung*. Oxford: Oxford University Press, 1994. Print.

Wolf, Sara. 'Sidi Larbi Cherkaoui's "Myth": The Choreographer, a Rising Star in Europe, Presents a U.S. Premiere at UCLA'. 2008. Web. Accessed: 22 October 2008 <http://www.latimes.com/news/nationworld/world/europe/la-et-myth20-2008oct20,0,885490.story>.

Ziolkowski, Jan. Ed. *Dante and Islam*. New York: Fordham University Press. 2014. Print.

Multimedia Source

Myth. Choreographed by Sidi Larbi Cherkaoui. 2007. Video Recording of Performance.

CHAPTER 7

Geopolitical Re-framing of the Nation and Language in *Babel*^(words)

Towards the end of this book and the decade of work created by Cherkaoui at the basis of this research, this chapter will work through key conclusions about the choreographer's negotiations of culture, nation and language as manifested in *Babel*^(words) (2010), co-choreographed by Cherkaoui and his long-term collaborator Damien Jalet. *Babel*^(words) marks a period of prolonged political impasse and federal instability in Belgium based on issues of language and territory. Typical of this fracturing state, Belgium's patchwork governance structure of overlapping communities and regions is characterised by devolution and centrifugality, rendering governmental decision-making increasingly problematic. Further detail about this complex federal structure and its implications was discussed in Chapter 1, the introduction to this book and then considered further in Chapter 2 with reference to Cherkaoui's first major choreographic work *Rien de Rien* (2000). In *Babel*^(words), these issues are refracted by bringing together 18 performers from 13 different countries, who express themselves in 15 different languages and represent 7 different religions. The questions of national identity, language and territory are reframed geopolitically on a global scale, away from the navel-gazing tendencies of recent political discourse in Belgian politics. *Babel*^(words) weaves together choreographic representations of borders, territories, shifting spaces and colliding identities. The two choreographers from opposite sides of the Belgian language border, reconsider the confounding of languages in the Old Testament not as a punishment but as an enriching cultural experience.

© The Author(s) 2019   175
L. Uytterhoeven, *Sidi Larbi Cherkaoui*, New World Choreographies,
https://doi.org/10.1007/978-3-030-27816-8_7

I spent a week in Antwerp witnessing the creation of *Babel*^(words) in July 2009, when workshops were held for a group of around 20 performers who had worked with Cherkaoui in the past or who were looking to collaborate with him in future productions. Some of the groundwork for *Babel*^(words) was laid in these workshops. The creation was then resumed in January until April 2010, with Lou Cope as dramaturg, with whom the connection was made a few years earlier when she observed the creative process of *Myth* (2007). I spent a week observing rehearsals in Brussels at the end of January and then another two weeks at the end of March and beginning of April. The production premiered on 27 April at the Cirque Royale in Brussels.

Babel^(words) is presented as the final part of a trilogy, after *Foi* (2003) and *Myth*. At the end of June and beginning of July 2010, these three works were presented in three consecutive weekends in Paris. The three main protagonists, Ulrika Kinn Svensson, Christine Leboutte and Darryl E. Woods, perform in these three productions. However, there is not a straightforward or linear narrative line connecting these three works. After *zero degrees* (co-choreographed with Akram Khan 2005) and *Sutra* (2008), this is the third Cherkaoui production which uses a set designed by Antony Gormley, and so it forms another kind of trilogy with those works. Musically, *Babel*^(words) is a transcultural encounter between two musicians from Patrizia Bovi's Italian Ensemble Micrologus, performing early music of the Mediterranean region, Japanese percussionist Shogo Yoshii from Kodo, and improvisers Mahabub and Sattar Khan from the Indian region of Rajasthan.

The starting point for Cherkaoui and Jalet's work was the Old Testament story of Babel: initially, there was only one language in the whole world. People decided they were going to build a tower that reached the heavens, not to worship God, but to make a name for themselves. Upon this arrogance, God descended and confounded the people's language so that they did not understand each other anymore. On the cover of Jalet's notebook used in the studio, there was an image of Pieter Bruegel the Elder's painting *The Tower of Babel* (c. 1563). In Chapter 6, a parallel was drawn between Cherkaoui's large group work *Myth*, the multiplicity of which resembles these late Medieval Flemish paintings. The image of the painting, physically brought into the creation space on the cover of the notebook, suggests the influence of late Medieval Flemish painting on the choreographic aesthetic. Like Bruegel's paintings and like previous large-group works by Cherkaoui, such as *Foi* and *Myth*, *Babel*^(words) is very full, busy, rich in imagery and multi-layered. The wealth of complex images in this work, like those that have come before, continues to present dramaturgical challenges for the spectator.

INTRODUCING BABEL^(WORDS) AS A GEOPOLITICAL WORK

The opening scene shows Svensson in a square of light reciting an excerpt from Nicole Krauss's fictional *The History of Love* (2006), explaining how in the Age of Silence, people communicated by gestures only, but they communicated more, not less. Misunderstandings were frequent, so people did not pretend they understood each other perfectly all the time. '[...] If at large gatherings or parties, or around people with whom you feel distant, your hands sometimes hang awkwardly at the ends of your arms – if you find yourself at a loss for what to do with them, overcome with sadness that comes when you recognize the foreignness of your own body – it's because your hands remember a time when the division between mind and body, brain and heart, what's inside and what's outside, was so much less. It's not like we've forgotten the language of gestures entirely. The habit of moving our hands when we speak is still left over from then. Clapping, pointing, giving the thumbs up, are all artefacts of ancient gestures. Holding hands, for example, is a way to remember what it feels like to say nothing, together. [...]'. Svensson combines reciting this text with a fabricated, repetitive sign language, which at times seems entirely dissonant with the content of her speech. For example, she includes the gesture flight attendants make when pointing out where the exits are on the plane, while the speech is not even remotely addressing that topic. Her expression is very plain and so is her intonation; she seems rather robotic. Futuristically dressed in shiny, black, plastic leggings, she resembles an artificial intelligence robot—a stark contrast to the hyper-human franticness she portrayed in *Foi* and *Myth*. This speech introduces important themes to the work and to Cherkaoui's oeuvre as a whole: communication (mis)understanding, connecting to others, the body, gestures, movements and touch.

The initial idea for *Babel*^(words) was that of cultural diversity. In a joint radio interview broadcast on national radio in April 2010, Cherkaoui and Jalet clarified that this idea stems from the artists' reality: 'as choreographers we encounter many people from different cultures, who express themselves in different languages. And still we find a common language within dance'. This seems to resonate with my reading of Cherkaoui's work as transcultural and cosmopolitan, in that he seeks to reveal what people have in common, rather than what sets them apart, and his utopian aim is to improve understanding between people (Olaerts). Jalet reveals that the subject of the work is 'the relationship between territory and language', which he considers 'an interesting theme for Belgium'. Jalet also explains: 'I speak French, he speaks Flemish; still we live in the same country. There is something that resonates for us in the subject of Babel'. This claim indicates that the production actively sought to address the then current political situation in Belgium, which had reached acute levels of impasse from 2007 to 2010. This situation resonates in the story of Babel, in which, Cherkaoui highlights, 'for the first time the blame is collective; therefore, in fact all people are guilty of pride'. The choreographers conclude that the story of Babel is an odd one, because it depicts cultural diversity as a punishment, while for them it is enriching. 'Maybe it can be a positive situation'.

One of the theoretical ideas underlying this production is that of geopolitics. While I was observing in January 2010, *Geopolitics: A Very Short Introduction* by Klaus Dodds was lying around on the table in the rehearsal studio. Geopolitics concerns itself with borders, territory and identities. The term is used in two very different ways: firstly, in its most commonly used form, it refers to 'a reliable guide of the global landscape using geographical descriptions, metaphors, and templates [...] It then helps to generate a simple model of the world, which can then be used to advise and inform foreign and security policy making' (Dodds 4). On the other hand, geopolitics can refer to the academic discipline that questions 'how geopolitics actually works' and 'particular understandings of places, communities, and accompanying identities' are generated (Dodds 5). These geopolitical developments are historically tainted by colonialism and global war. In *Babel^(words)* ideas of territory, communication and border checkpoints are choreographed in various ways, indicating that the work is intensely concerned with and seeks to foreground geopolitics. In which ways are geopolitical ideas of place, community and identity relevant to the broader political context in which Cherkaoui creates work? In particular, what is the impact of Belgium as a fracturing state on conceptions of national identity, as choreographically negotiated by Cherkaoui? These will be the questions explored in the next sections. However, due to its multi-layered and complex composition and dramaturgy, the work also enables a parallel to be drawn between the engaged spectatorship that it invites and the hermeneutic nature of critical geopolitics itself.

Returning to the analysis of *Babel*$^{(words)}$, ideas of territory and its relationship to national identity are introduced choreographically in a scene at the beginning of the performance, which the performers refer to as 'The Line'. The dancers sit on their knees next to each other. Their hands rest on their legs, then slide down to the floor and when their fingertips reach the floor, they slide their hands out to the side until they meet the next person's wrist. Each dancer says the word 'land' in their own language, as if they are laying claim on this land as their own territory: 'terre', 'earth', 'al 'ard', 'jord', 'land', etc. Yoshii's sharp, irregular, percussive rhythms on a small drum meticulously correspond to the sharp borders the dancers trace with their fingertips in the space around them, all moving in precise unison. Space is delineated, measured, swapped and pushed to the side. Borders are drawn, quickly erased and re-drawn. Eyes follow the fingertips' movements and occasionally cast a threatening look on a neighbour who is coming a bit too close. The tempo speeds up. When the dancers get to their feet, they move as if they were stuck inside an invisible box, still maintaining the unison between them. Entrenched in their own little space—or nation state—they bang their elbows, knees and heads against these invisible walls. 'Duets', or fights, start to form, in which each dancer bashes into their neighbour. The multitude of synchronous duets serves the idea that these kinds of struggles over territory are not unique, but happening in multiple places around the world at the same time. The duets turn into trios. The shapes made by the dancing bodies slot into one another perfectly as each thrust comes to a finish. Power is rotated between the dancers with every blow, without anyone coming out victorious. Then, it becomes a fight between six dancers. The more bodies become involved in the fight, the more complex the composition. Three of the frames are drawn into the light and provide a more delineated space in which the staccato fighting, the constant issuing of blows—less and less discriminate about who is on the receiving end of them—between dancers continues. These frames are pushed together in an intricate formation, like the tectonic plates at the basis of the earth's continents, although in a direction opposite to continental drift.

The cube is at the centre of the frame formation and all the dancers gather inside. The space is crowded, and to the sound of a ticking time bomb, they shove and tug each other around, each trying to push to the front. To the loud blows of the drum, one dancer at a time jumps out of the cube from one pose to the next, a string of dancers travelling around through the other frames and beyond, colonising the space around them. The three protagonists, Svensson, Woods and Leboutte, are left standing in the cube. Woods is in the centre, wearing a light grey suit, and clearly holds the most power. Leboutte is dressed in a gipsy-like loose dress and her hairstyle is messy. Svensson still has a robotic appearance to her, although she was functioning perfectly well among the humans. Paea Leach finishes the staccato thrusting downstage, reverting back to the initial hand and wrist movements from 'The Line'.

The harp rapidly plays scale after scale to signal a change of atmosphere to a more light-hearted dream scenario. In the next scene, space is detached from the concept of the nation state, becomes less about geography and is reframed as a commodity which is desired, bought and sold. Woods opens his arms and says 'Welcome' in a charming voice, before launching into an elaborate real estate sales pitch for his 'spatial concept adapted to your urban living needs'. The frame formation to which he gestures has become a luxury penthouse apartment and is described as 'functional, stark, modular' and benefitting from not only 'striking geometry' but also 'convertability'. Whisking the audience in with his finger, he says 'Let's move on', before flamboyantly turning around and strutting through a narrow corridor with his hands thrown into the air triumphantly. Speaking like an estate agent, he mentions the Golden Ratio and the Fibonacci sequence with reference to—said in a soft, sexy voice—the space's 'organic inevitability', as he slides up and down the edge of one of the frames as if he is pole dancing. As he moves through the space, his force field pushes Leboutte out of the way. She looks uneasy and clumsy in the space and starts to clean it. Woods references Ancient Chinese beliefs while putting his palms together and bowing, as we hear a stereotypically Asian tune on a string instrument. Bringing his sales pitch to an end, Woods throws in some empty-sounding numbers about the economy, the Dow Jones, the Nasdaq and the FTSE-100, to highlight what a great opportunity this is to buy. 'It's high-instinct, high-cost, high-profit, high-impact and – best of all – it's high-up!' He invites us to 'sign on the dotted line' and all this could be ours. 'Remember, it's hard to be down, when you're up!', he says in *glissando* voice, his thumbs rising upwards. This scene introduces the idea that, while emotional arguments about the

nation state are often on the surface about territory, an underlying capitalist agenda tends to dictate geopolitical developments more or less invisibly.
The inception and creation of *Babel*$^{(words)}$ coincided with the 2008
global economic crisis, which drew attention to the pitfalls of capitalism
and neoliberal policies. Exposing levels of inequality caused by capitalism and how their degree of power proscribes how people are invited to
inhabit different spaces, Leboutte has got down on her knees, cleaning
the floor. She hesitantly sings a traditional song, verse by verse, as her
voice grows more and more weepy. Svensson trots in, her arms held stiff
by her sides, but her shoulders and head bopping from side to side as she
walks. Other dancers come in and surround Leboutte, whose singing has
now become more like shouting, as she hits her hand flat on the ground.
They efficiently slide the frame away and her with it, erasing her presence
and rendering her labour invisible.

Svensson has collapsed down on the floor, her arms in an awkward
angle. Kazutimo Kozuki and Yoshii advance towards her, speaking
Japanese between them. As soon as he spots her, Kozuki shouts 'Ooh
ooh ooh, Ulrika, Ulrika', but Yoshii does not seem to understand what
the fuss is about. 'Scandinavia, Sweden, uh, Ikea!', Kozuki explains,
reversing the stereotyping that Europeans tend to do about Asian culture. He turns an imaginary knob on the back of her head and 'switches
her on'. He presses a pretend button on her back and she opens and
closes the fingers on her left hand repeatedly. Next, she bends and
stretches her arm, while turning her head left and right, and vacantly
smiling and losing the smile, repeatedly. He yanks an imaginary wire at
the back and she starts moving her head in a circular motion, while waving her hand. Then, she seems out of control, and they 'reboot' her by
switching her off and on again. She accidentally punches Kozuki in the
face. They make whizzing and beeping sounds to accompany her movements and seem fascinated at what she can do. Holding her hand, he
blows onto one of her fingers and she rises from her knees to standing,
while her cheeks are rounded with air. Already quite literally objectified
as a sexy robot in skin-tight PVC trousers that trots vacuously around
the stage, she has now become a veritable sex doll. The two grab a
hand each and sing a Japanese song into it like a microphone or karaoke
machine.

Later in the work, the aluminium structures are arranged in a diagonal corridor and the performers enact a border checkpoint situation. The
performers are split into two groups, contained in two of the structures

on either side of the corridor. Woods and Svensson stand in the middle. Woods invites Jon Filip Fahlstrøm to come through the corridor, saying 'Next!' in a matter of fact voice. He asks: 'Did you pack your bags yourself? Is that a weapon of mass destruction in your pocket, or are you just happy to see me?' Svensson swipes her forearms horizontally from one side to the other, leading the way through the corridor, while curtseying and tilting her head and wishing Fahlstrøm a pleasant journey in Swedish, in a robotic, fake-friendly way. Navala Chaudhari hands Svensson an imaginary passport, which the latter moves downwards in front of her face, scanning its content. Woods inquires whether she is 'carrying any drugs or alcohol, Madam? Hiding anything in between your tits [as he looks inside her cleavage]? Hash in your ass?' Svensson brings an end to this inquisition by leading Chaudhari through the corridor and saying in the poshest English voice possible, 'Have a pleasant journey'. Next, Kozui and Yoshii are up to be inspected. Scanning their imaginary passports, Svensson beeps to indicate an error. The two Japanese men start talking rapidly between themselves and at the two border officials. Svensson responds by speaking gibberish back in a Japanese accent. Scanning the passport again, without problems this time, the two men are ushered through. Bovi is next, and Woods inquires whether she is carrying any mozzarella or is a member of the Mafia. Svensson invites her to go through with a greeting in Italian. When Mohamed Benaji and Moya Michael, who has wrapped a scarf around her head, try to go through, Svensson already begins beeping to indicate a problem long before any passports are scanned. Woods asks her to remove her headscarf, and Benaji speaks for her, in Arabic, presumably explaining that she is not allowed to remove it in public. Again, Svensson responds in gibberish with an Arabic accent and gestures towards her face, as if explicating that they need to be able to see Michael's face. Cherkaoui mentioned during the creation that Svensson's response was inspired by a comedy sketch from the Catherine Tate show, called '*The Offensive Translator*' on YouTube, in which Tate steps in for an absent translator for a UN meeting in the most incompetent and offensive way, reducing the languages and cultures of the people around the table to the easiest possible stereotypes. In the scene, crucially, Benaji and Michael are permitted to go through. When the gipsy-like Leboutte tries to go through, Svensson immediately starts to beep again. Leboutte tries to sneak past, but Svensson grabs her collar and pulls her back again. She leads her to the side, where she pats her down in a polite and professional, but increasingly invasive manner. She moves her fingers in front of Leboutte's face to scan her facial features and retina, but then also prods her finger in Leboutte's ear. She pulls open Leboutte's jaw and looks inside her mouth like an animal. She stands behind Leboutte and cups her breasts in her hands, lifting and releasing the breasts one by one. She sticks her hands inside Leboutte's neckline and rummages around in her clothing. Spreading Leboutte's arms and legs apart, Svensson does the same between her legs underneath her skirt. Leboutte looks unhappy but entirely powerless to stop the examination. Finally, Svensson invites Leboutte to go through to the other side, wishing her 'Un bon voyage'. However, Leboutte says, first in French and then in English, that she prefers to stay where she is. As this lack of compliance is messing up the system, Svensson gets stuck repeating the phrase 'Un bon, un bon, un bon, un bon voy-voy-voy-voyage' and starts mixing in her gibberish Japanese and Arabic, as she stumbles away. Leboutte sings an *a capella* traditional song, while the other performers harmonise with her inside one of the structures that is being slid around the stage. They eventually subsume her and lead her away in their vehicle. This is the second time that Leboutte's undesired presence is cleared away by the others. Accompanied by Bovi's solo singing, Svensson then lets her joints collapse, knees and elbows turned in, limbs folding in and unfolding in rapid succession as if her movements are stuck in a loop, while she stutters a few phrases of the Krauss text she spoke at the beginning of the work. Towards the end of her solo, she stutters the phrase 'Forgive me', but it quickly becomes 'Give me, give me, give me', as she extends her arm forward and opens and closes the upturned palm of her hand.

In one of the metal structures turned onto its long side, Francis Ducharme loftily pontificates about how Svensson's solo is a prime example of Belgian contemporary dance in which words are added to the dance, common since the 1980s. As he walks through the frame, he takes off his suit jacket to reveal a fur sleeveless jacket and bends down, stops talking, and imitates a primate's movements, arms dangling over the floor. This caveman takes an interest in Svensson, soon turning sexual. She barely moves but is able to flick him away with just a small movement of the wrist. She sits down in mermaid pose, both legs turned to one side, and the growling caveman approaches her in a way that resembles the wolf-like duets between her and Jalet in *Myth*. Again, she pushes him away. He returns to make a grunt, up close to her face, and the sound 'echoes' in her empty body, as Svensson repeats the grunts three or four times, softer each time. A few grunts later, instead of vocalising the echo, Svensson answers with 'I am not afraid of tomorrow, for I have seen yesterday and I love today', a quote from William Allen White about which the spectator may be unsure what its significance is. She hypnotises Ducharme by rapidly circling her index finger in front of his face, then sticks her finger up his nose and throws him to the side. She sticks her finger under her armpit and twists it a few times to clean it. Ducharme hops back sideways through the frame, getting a bit higher with each hop, picks up his jacket and casually throws it over his shoulder when he has 'evolved' back into modern man. He whisks her over, but she does not come. Eventually, he says in French that it seems as if they no longer manage to communicate and he wants to take a break in their relationship and take some time to think.

Babel$^{(words)}$ thus continues to work through some of the key dramaturgical issues that marked Cherkaoui's oeuvre during the 2000–2010 period from a geopolitical perspective. The issues of the nation and national identity are played out through the drawing of borders and representing what happens when different people move across these borders. An interrogation of language and translation is developed both through the performers' use of their native languages and the focus on the role of gestures in non-verbal communication in Svensson's speech. Moreover, a trace of the notion of the offensive translator already features in Kozuki and Yoshii's Japanese scene, with which those who do not speak the language are necessarily limited to having only a rudimentary, stereotypical engagement. This is enacted by the offensive robotic translator played by Svensson later at the border crossing, perhaps confirming the spectator's own worst fears about the limits of understanding across cultural borders. These painful notions are couched in Jalet and Cherkaoui's bittersweet humour, which helps to reopen the possibilities of communication. Humour also characterises Cherkaoui and Jalet's continued self-reflexive examination of dance history in the scene between Ducharme and Svensson. As suggested in Chapter 2, the unease with which Cherkaoui refers to dance historical developments in, for example, Marie-Louise Wilderijkx's solo in *Rien de Rien* indicates a sense of exclusion from and unease with that history from Cherkaoui's postcolonial perspective. In *Babel*$^{(words)}$, however, Ducharme and Svensson's self-reflexive scene also highlights the wider limits of certain forms of contemporary dance that are posited as elitist in terms of their ability to effectuate social change, which is what Cherkaoui's dramaturgical strategies aim to do. What is new in *Babel*(words), for the first time in the decade of Cherkaoui's work that is the focus of this book, is a more explicit focus on economic inequality in the wake of the 2008 global financial crisis, through highlighting the contrast between Woods and Leboutte in the apartment sales pitch scene. Leboutte subsequent dire treatment at the border crossing indicates how this inequality also has an impact on people's mobility.

ALTERNATIVE MODERNITIES

In addition to snippets of spoken text from Krauss and the estate agent's sales pitch, *Babel*(words) continues Cherkaoui's creative exploration of storytelling. In his works, Cherkaoui can increasingly be seen to be tapping into a whole new resource of orally transmitted material, namely that which is made available online via YouTube or TED. In *Apocrifu* (2007), an excerpt of a YouTube speech is recited and choreographed. This was fully discussed in Chapter 4 in terms of its religious implications. In *Babel*(words), after a comic scene in which they are manipulated like robots, Svensson and Fahlstrøm face each other and perform gestural actions on each other's torso, as if they are programming each other like a robot in reference to a previous scene in *Babel*(words). The musicians reproduce a tune, originally by electronic music duo Fischerspooner, acoustically on their instruments. They then turn to face someone else and the programming gradually multiplies until there is a diagonal line of face-to-face duets, in which the dancers perform and repeat a movement sequence extending and rotating their arms, hands and fingers, as if they are turning knobs and pressing buttons on each other's torso. Leboutte manoeuvres between them, trying to clean them, but struggling, because their arms move too quickly. They then face the audience and continue to programme the immediate space around them. Benaji transforms these movements into locking and popping, as he moves across the stage. After a while Woods, dressed in a nerdy gilet and wearing thick-rimmed glasses, walks downstage and addresses the audience. He recites the 2009 online TED lecture 'The Neurons that Shaped Civilization' by neuroscientist Vilayanur Ramachandran, which has been widely disseminated on social networks. He explains how mirror neurons function and allow us to imitate and learn complex social behaviour, which can be seen as the basis for human culture. He argues that we are able to empathise when we watch another person being touched, and that it is our skin that prevents us from becoming confused in that we know we are not actually being touched.

'Now it turns out there are neurons that are called ordinary motor command neurons in the front of the brain, which have been known for over 50 years. These neurons will fire, when a person performs a specific action. [...] but it has also been found that a subset of these neurons, maybe about 20% of them, will also fire when I'm looking at somebody else performing the same action. So, here's a neuron that fires when I reach and grab something, but it also fires when I watch Joe reaching and grabbing something and this is truly astonishing because it is as though this neuron is adopting the other person's point of view. It is almost as if it is performing a virtual reality simulation of the other person's action. Now what is the significance of these mirror neurons? For one thing, they must be involved in things like imitation and emulation. Because to imitate a complex act, it requires your brain to adopt the other person's point of view, and this is how learning happens, and once an action is learned it spreads in geometric proportion across the population. This is what we call culture; this is the basis of civilization. Now, there is another kind of mirror neuron, which is involved in something quite different and that is: there are mirror neurons systems. There are mirror neurons for actions; there are mirror neurons for touch. In other words, if somebody touches me on my hand, a neuron in the somatosensory cortex, in the sensory region of the brain, fires. But the same neuron in some cases will fire when I simply watch another person being touched, so it's empathizing the other person being touched. Now the question then arises, if I simply watch another person being touched, why do I not get confused and literally feel that touch sensation? Well that's because you've got receptors in your skin, touch and pain receptors, going back into your brain and saying, "don't worry, you're not being touched", so empathize by all means with the other person but do not actually experience the touch, otherwise you'll get confused and muddled. But if you remove the arm, you simply anesthetize my arm, so you put an injection in my arm and anesthetize the brachial plexus so the arm is numb and there are no sensations coming in... If I now watch you being touched, I literally feel it in my hand. In other words, you've dissolved the barrier between you and other human beings. All that's separating you from him, from the other person is your skin. Remove the skin, you experience that person's touch in your mind. You have dissolved the barrier between you and other human beings and this, of course, is the basis of much of Eastern Philosophy and that is, there is no real independent self, aloof from other human beings, inspecting the world and inspecting other people. You are in fact connected not just via Facebook and the internet. You're actually quite literally connected by your neurons and there's whole chains of neurons around this room talking to each other, and there is no real distinctiveness of your conscious from somebody else's conscious. And this is not just mumbo-jumbo philosophy; it emerges from our understanding of basic neuroscience'.

In this scene, there is a striking similarity between the gestural programming actions performed by the dancers and the gestural body language performed by Woods, who has copied Ramachandran's movements exactly from the online video. Predictably, towards the end of the text, the other dancers join Woods in performing Ramachandran's gestural body language—except Svensson who keeps robotically performing the programming gestures, indicating that she is not human as she is not moving under the influence of these mirror neurons. This scene is a continuation and development of Cherkaoui's interest in unison storytelling since *Rien de Rien* and *zero degrees* (2005). Here, Cherkaoui and Jalet present communication—spoken language and body language—as something humans are technologically programmed to do in a specific way. In a broader sense, they seem to propose that, in line with Butler's performativity and Foucauldian notions of a disciplined body, identity is performed under the influence of discourse. Afterwards, Helder Seabra and Michael perform a duet starting with their fingertips walking over each other's skin, first in the cube, then beyond it. Michael had already broken free from the rigidity of the programming during the previous scene, moving freely through the group by going off balance and following these impulses through sequentially in the rest of her body. Michael and Seabra gently explore each other's body, lifting and supporting each other. Bovi slowly and tentatively plays the harp and gently sings. When watching this duet, I feel my skin tingle, Woods/Ramachandran's words echoing in my mind. Hence, the use of the spoken word enhanced my affective engagement with the choreography.

While the travel stories in Cherkaoui's works, discussed in Chapter 3 in the context of transculturality in *zero degrees*, point towards his interest in travel, migration, displacement and destabilised identities, in the sense that these are elements that enrich one's life and need to be celebrated, the stories taken from the Internet indicate a sensitivity towards the worldwide availability of stories through digital online media. According to Arjun Appadurai, both these mechanisms work to erode national boundaries and the imagined, uncomplicated national identities that were constructed during Western modernity and the Enlightenment. Appadurai argues that the current globalised world demands news concepts, approaches and critical discourses in order to make sense of a deterritorialised world that is no longer neatly delineated by nations and cultures tied to specific places. He considers the impact of migration and the media on how the modern world is imagined, and on identity, which becomes more and more unstable and less reliant on the concept of the nation state. Instead, Appadurai introduces a set of five neologisms, based on adding the suffix '-scape': 'ethnoscapes', 'mediascapes', 'technoscapes', 'financescapes' and 'ideoscapes'. These scapes can be considered as complex, flowing and overlapping building blocks that can be used to imagine the modern world, in favour of fixed landscapes. Of these five 'imagined worlds' (Appadurai 33), ethnoscapes, mediascapes and ideoscapes are the most relevant to Cherkaoui's choreographic oeuvre.

Cherkaoui's world view seems heavily influenced by the idea of travelling in line with Appadurai's focus on 'ethnoscape', or

> the landscape of persons who constitute the shifting world in which we live: tourists, immigrants, refugees, exiles, guest workers, and other moving groups and individuals constitute an essential feature of the world and appear to affect the politics of (and between) nations to a hitherto unprecedented degree. (Appadurai 33)

Cherkaoui, the son of a displaced Moroccan guest labourer in Flanders, seeks to surround himself with performers and collaborators who, like him, have stories to tell of displacement, which is then actively explored through verbal and corporeal storytelling in his work. He particularly foregrounds the travel story as a site where cultures clash in the 'contact zone', in Pratt's terms. From analysis of geopolitical works like *zero degrees* and *Babel*$^{(words)}$, it is clear that Cherkaoui underwrites Appadurai's theorisation of the erosion of the nation state and national identity as a consequence of migration and other human movement across the planet. Contrary to Appadurai, however, Cherkaoui does not understand this as a recent phenomenon limited to the last few decades, but on many occasions has emphasised that people have travelled already for thousands of years preceding the creation of the nation state and drawn attention to the cultural evidence of this migration and transcultural exchange, which he includes in his choreographies.

With mediascapes, Appadurai draws attention to the electronic production and dissemination of information through the mass, broadcast and post-broadcast media. The term also includes the 'large and complex repertoires of images, narratives, and ethnoscapes' created by these mediascapes (Appadurai 35). While different kinds of media representing the world have been in use for thousands of years, it could be argued that especially the World Wide Web—which had not yet come to full fruition at the time Appadurai was writing—has transformed the perception of the world for masses of people in the last two decades. Instant communication, including the exchange of images and texts, is now possible with someone who is miles away. Vast quantities of texts, images and films are only a mouse-click away, free and immediately accessible. Appadurai argues that the world views which ensue in the imagination from these mediascapes are distorted because of a blurring of reality and fiction. This, in turn, has an influence on how the Other is perceived. Cherkaoui's tentative use of material available from the Internet indicates his interest in the potential of mediascapes. He taps into these messy repertoires of images and stories, brought to the creation through the performers' personal experiences or through the exploration of online material. Appadurai argues that mediascapes are adapted and compiled by people into more coherent wholes:

> Mediascapes [...] tend to be image-centred, narrative-based accounts of strips of reality, and what they offer to those who experience and transform them is a series of elements (such as characters, plots, and textual forms) out of which scripts can be formed of imagined lives, their own as well as those of others living in other places. (Appadurai 35)

Cherkaoui's works consist similarly of image-centred, narrative-based fragments, and function for the spectator in a similar way as Appadurai's mediascapes. Spectators engaging with Cherkaoui's work also transform it into imagined wholes, yet each of them does so differently. However, while Cherkaoui mimics the workings of mediascapes in his works, he also departs from these as unspoken and uncritical doings, by placing the stories told in his works under increased scrutiny through the spectator's affective engagement. His choreographic strategies of duplication, distortion and disruption play tricks on the spectator and invite a more

critical, questioning stance as part of the continuous spectatorial dramaturgy. A more intent listening happens through the vocal and corporeal
treatment Cherkaoui gives these stories, raising questions about whose
stories these are and why they are told in the ways they are, as part of the
continuous dramaturgy of the spectator.

Ideoscapes refer to political and ideological 'chain[s] of ideas, terms,
and images' that consist of elements of the Enlightenment worldview,
including 'freedom, welfare, rights, sovereignty, representation, and [...]
democracy' (Appadurai 36). However, the diaspora of these ideoscapes
puts them under increased pressure of mistranslation in the diverging
contexts in which they have been appropriated. He finds it problematic,
in the context of 'ideoscapes', that the ideology and world view of the
Enlightenment have undergone a worldwide diaspora, but have become
detached from the internal logic of its original context. Hence, this
Western ideology has been appropriated incompletely and become lost
in translation. Therefore, Appadurai seems to allude to the limitations of
a continued use of this set of ideas as 'correct'. The interest in oral histories and storytelling, and the distrust of the written word in history and
religion, indicate that Cherkaoui, in line with Appadurai, is sensitive to
those kinds of postcolonial and postmodern critiques. In a broader sense,
the use of narration in Cherkaoui's works prompts a re-evaluation of the
configuration of writing and speech in Western society. Cherkaoui's choreographic engagement with Appadurai's ideoscapes was discussed in
more detail in Chapter 4 with regard to religious fundamentalism and
Cherkaoui's choreographic negotiations thereof.

In sum, a parallel can be drawn between Cherkaoui's choreographic
inclusion of stories from many different perspectives and different parts
of the world and anthropological and ethnographic practices which
favour individual voices and the particular. These writing practices share
with Cherkaoui a common interest in a destabilised sense of Self resulting from mixed cultural identity or migration. However, stories are continually presented as shared by more than one body and in the case of
Ramachandran's online lecture in $Babel^{(words)}$ by a chorus of performers.
Here, through the increased visual impact of the corporeal multiplication,
Cherkaoui and Jalet may be inviting the audience to share in the stories as
well and consider their content more intently. The choreographic treatment of the stories through various strategies thus has implications for
spectatorship and the configuration of perception in the theatre, as well as
the continuous dramaturgical engagement of the spectator.

In his works, Cherkaoui addresses aspects of cultural modernity in relation to the forcible construction of identity through exclusionary social categories, such as nationality, religion, race and gender, and the role of the written word in establishing and perpetuating such social categories. He counteracts this modernity through the inclusion of storytelling and through dramaturgical exploration of historiographical processes. Unlike Walter Benjamin's apparent longing for a pre-modern state of being in 'The Storyteller', a mythical and undefined past, Cherkaoui draws from the reality of his own professional situation, which is based on transnational collaboration and transcultural exchange, and seems to operate in a kind of 'modernity at large' (Appadurai), one that is worldwide and uncontrollable.

CIRCUMAMBULATING THE CONTINUOUS TRANSFORMATION OF SPACE

The visual design of *Babel*^(*words*) invites a further linking of Appadurai's fluid and shifting-scapes to the work's geopolitical dramaturgy. Through their choreographic interaction with Gormley's metallic frames, the performers are able to create a wide range of meanings about space and the ways in which it can include and exclude people. In one key scene towards the start of the work, Seabra is caught in one of the frames, which acts as a prison. Accompanied by ominous-sounding, low humming voices and beats of the drum responsively timed to his movements, Seabra bangs his shoulders, elbows and head against the imagined walls of his prison cell, to no avail, until he drops down on the floor exhausted. This movement sequence may be seen as a reference to Michel Foucault's *Discipline and Punish*. The frames are transparent; there are no walls. The audience can see into people's homes at the back of the stage, so there is a panoptic element about these frames, making them ideal for observation and surveillance. The boundaries of public and private space are blurred, like in Lars von Trier's film *Dogville* (2003), a film Cherkaoui had mentioned to me before, in which people's houses have no walls but there are only lines on the floor. Through the ways in which the performers behave in, and hence give meaning to, the spaces created by the different configurations of Gormley's metallic structures, the spectator may become aware of the hypervisibility of what goes on inside the frames, thus alluding to the effects of CCTV and

data surveillance in the twenty-first century. In *Babel*^(words), the walls of
the prison are not only transparent, but also selectively permeable, as is
demonstrated by a passer-by drifting into the cell and out again.

Gormley's set design plays a crucial role in the dramaturgy of
Babel^(words), and therefore, it is necessary to describe and analyse the
design on its own as well as in relation to the choreography. On one of
my first visits in January 2010, Cherkaoui exclaimed: 'This is our set!'
pointing to a scale model on top of the grand piano in the rehearsal studio. They would have to wait for the full scale set to arrive in the rehearsal
studio until mid-February 2010. Gormley designed five cuboid frames
of various dimensions, including one cube, made out of aluminium alloy.
While the different shapes of the boxes create the illusion that one box is
larger than another, the volume of the five boxes is equal by approxima-
tion. The implication here is that it is not always possible to trust one's
eye and intuitive judgements about something, like in a game of optical
illusion. During rehearsals, Cherkaoui would often demonstrate what he
would like to achieve by manipulating the model while the performers
joined him around the piano. This is not a new approach, given that the
scale model of Gormley's set for *Sutra* found its way into the work itself,
manipulated by Cherkaoui and Dong Dong at the start of the work as if
they are playing a game of chess. During the creation of *Babel*^(words), the
performers then tried the manipulations modelled by Cherkaoui with the
full-size frames and grew very skilled at moving and tilting the structures
around safely and economically, cooperating with each other as necessary.
The cube is designed to be climbable, although the performers climb
some of the other structures too. When the longest structure is put on
its side so that it stands tall, it does not give the impression of being very
stable. Likewise, the longer sides of the structures bend down when they
bear weight. I remember feeling rather uncomfortable at the pliability
of the material, as I experienced this as an imperfection. The structures
are so shiny and perfectly symmetrical that I was expecting them to also
be rigid and reliable. Some of the performers tended to stretch out their
shoulders by hanging from the sides of the structure. I felt myself wanting to tell them that they should not do this on the longer sides of the
structures, as it made them droop slightly, which I perceived as unpleas-
ant to the eye. However, these tensions between the stark, angular aesthetics of the frames and the reality of the pliability of the material are just
one of the ways in which the choreographic interactions with the design
implicate the spectator on an affective level (Fig. 7.1).

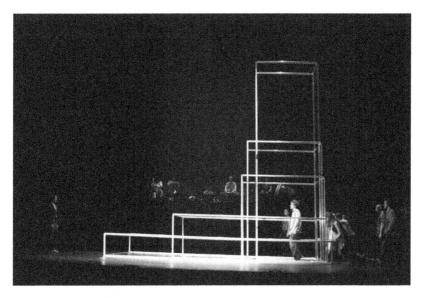

Fig. 7.1 *Babel*$^{(words)}$ by Sidi Larbi Cherkaoui and Damien Jalet (Photo by Koen Broos)

Reflecting semiologically on the meanings associated with aluminium alloy, it is a material which has been crucial as a building material in construction and transportation since the late Industrial Revolution. It has also become an important material in modern domestic life, most notably due to its lightness and pliability. For example, drink cans, foil and foil trays are made out of aluminium and can be recycled. Aluminium must be extracted from the natural materials in the earth's crust using an electrolysis process in order to exist in a usable form, a process which consumes a lot of energy. The smelting process requires a lot of electricity and therefore tends to happen in locations where electricity is plentiful and inexpensive, for example South Africa, Australia, China and Canada (Schmitz, Domagala & Haag 27). These areas of the world are relatively newly industrialised, raising the question of where materials widely used in modern Western life come from and what the human and ecologic cost of their production is. It can also be noted that the Industrial Revolution in Europe roughly coincided with the birth and development of the nation state and national identity. The use of the alloy in Gormley's designs may be a deliberate invitation for the spectator to reflect on the wider historical context in which the geopolitical shaping of modern Europe and the world occurred.

In *Babel*$^{(words)}$, throughout the performance, the performers frequently drag the five structures across the floor into new formations. To Bovi's gentle plucking of the harp, they tilt the structures away from each other, then all together simultaneously to stage left, then upstage, except for one which is tilted downstage. This contrast emphasises the structures' three-dimensionality, as the light glistens on the metal frames. They pivot the structures around and gently slide them into new places. They manipulate them in such a way that they create different shapes and architectural forms. Joined together in a diamond floor pattern with the lowest structure at the front and tallest at the back, the structures resemble a Gothic cathedral. The performers walk around inside, gawking at the architecture, their gaze slightly directed upwards. Standing outside the cathedral, they then pull the structures outward, so that it resembles an opening lotus flower, echoing a similar image from *Sutra*, in which Gormley's wooden boxes were manipulated in much the same way. Now, the metallic structures are flat and low, and the sense of space is completely transformed. A few tilts later, the structures are pushed together into a cross formation on the floor with the cube at the centre. Immediately, the cross begins to rotate on the floor, so that it then resembles an elaborate, futuristic spaceship. Kozuki walks inside to the edges of one of the spaceship's wings, while pretending to turn knobs and push buttons all around him. Michael travels up and down the wing created by the structure that is the narrowest, which is on its narrow side. Her movements emphasise this narrowness, as she swings her arms back and forth close to her body. Leach has more space to dance around in her wing, so she turns with arms extended. As the spaceship keeps rotating, Kozuki, Michael and Leach have to continuously and carefully keep treading sideways to avoid getting their toes stuck underneath the moving metal structures, as well as concentrate on travelling outwards to the edges of the spaceship's wings and back towards its centre. The spaceship then comes to a halt.

Other instruments and voices join in to create an intricate musical landscape. The narrowest structure is tilted onto its broadside, and Ducharme rolls around inside it. The cube is tilted and slid into the other structure over its edge. The performers have to cooperate to make this happen, walking their hands up and down the frames, one lowering the cube on one side, the other standing on the opposite side, providing counterweight to ensure the cube is lowered in a controlled manner. Benaji breakdances inside the cube, as another structure is slid over the cube and inside the first structure. Next, a fourth structure is added to the construction, tipped over the edge of the cube and lowered inside. The cube and this other, slightly taller and narrower structure are then tipped, so that they rest diagonally on the edges of another structure. This way, the final structure can be lowered inside more easily, as it is very long. Benaji dances on an increasingly smaller patch of ground on the very inside of the formation. With this tall structure now fully erect, all the performers have to do is push it centre stage and centre all the structures perfectly one inside the other. Seabra is standing awestruck at the centre of this tower and sits down cross-legged in a meditating position. The tower slowly spins around him.

These constantly shifting images, creating diverging, multiple meanings bear resemblance with a key scene in *Myth*, where the symbol of the cross was circumambulated, wandering in front of the eye of the spectator, and different layers of meaning were excavated as a kind of dreamwork. This was discussed in more detail in Chapter 6. In *Babel*$^{(words)}$, because the imagery works affectively on the spectator through the scene's non-verbality, calm music and slow-moving actions, a space of reflection is created to let these different layers of meaning sink in and to link different fragments of the dramaturgy together. The architecture that the performers create comes to metaphorically stand for all things man-made—that is, culture—which can, on the one hand, be very beautiful, impressive, touching and on the other hand, arrogant, having caused division between people through enforcing exclusionary social categories.

The whole tower is tipped back in its entirety, using all the strength of the workforce to do this in a controlled manner. Seabra has got to his feet and comes out from underneath, pulling the central, tall structure along with him, until it juts out perfectly symmetrically on both sides. This new formation is also spun around gently, now with James O'Hara at the centre. O'Hara then exits the structure and dances freely on the stage space next to it, spinning endlessly and spiralling down to the floor and back up again, echoing the previous spinning of the structures. Next the structures are dragged to the back to resemble a city skyline. The performers embark on a highly structured walking sequence, tracing geometrical patterns on the floor. They are all walking in a rapid, busy and determined fashion. At the back, Woods is pacing up and down inside the narrow structure, talking busily into a pretend mobile phone. Leach and O'Hara dance a duet amidst this rigid and busy activity, tumbling on top of each other and rolling on the floor while holding hands.

The pace picks up as the structures are spun and dragged along the floor at high speed in the 'Running Structures' scene, where performers run, jump and roll in and out and over and under the edges of the frames. It is an exhilarating scene, in which the performers are seeking out thrills and an adrenaline rush, much like a rollercoaster. When watching this scene be created, I feared for people's toes. Some performers wore trainers, and others were barefoot. Seabra explained to me that his choice to be barefoot stems from the fact that he trusts his bare feet more than he trusts shoes (Seabra). The effect of apparent danger in moving between the structures barefoot was not deliberate, but an added bonus to help the spectators, now confronted with the unease of seeing toes nearly stubbed and performers nearly tripping, to become affectively connected to the actions and present realities of the performers. The cube is even tipped onto one of its corners while being spun, and Benaji responds by jumping in and out over its edges. O'Hara clambers on top of another structure, which is also being spun, and sits on top of it, surveying the action. Ducharme lies face down on the floor inside one structure, his arms extended and grabbing on to the edges of the frame, while it is still being spun. Seabra spins around alternately taking his weight onto his hands and feet. Damien Fournier, Benaji and Fahlstrøm traverse the stage one by one, jumping, doing backflips and breakdancing. Meanwhile, Leboutte has draped washing lines with clothes hanging from them onto another structure. This is now being dragged across the stage too, like a caravan, while she dances inside in an exuberant, gipsy-like manner and plays castanets. All five structures are now being moved around, but it is not long before the thrill-seeking ends in a huge collision of two structures crashing head-on (Fig. 7.2).

The consequence of the desire to move Gormley's cuboid structures and continually transform the space through the different configurations that the frames make is that the group of performers has to work closely together to make these movements possible. The physical reality of the frames, their size and weight, combined with the effects of gravity, means that cooperation between the performers is necessary to make the structures move safely and smoothly. This sense of cooperation appears

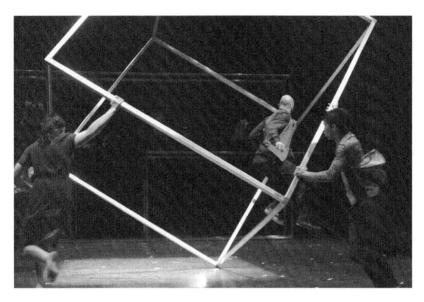

Fig. 7.2   Paea Leach, Mohamed Benaji and Jon Filip Fahlstrøm in *Babel^(words)* (Photo by Koen Broos)

to be a larger geopolitical metaphor, standing for what is needed to enable humanity to survive and live together on this planet. This could be related back to the Bible story of Babel, in which people worked together to build the tower and hence make a name for themselves. In Cherkaoui and Jalet's *Babel^(words)*, in contrast, people revert back to the first language of the body to communicate with each other, before the biblical confusion of languages and manage to cooperate beautifully. Although the smooth and efficient manipulation of the frames is carefully choreographed and rehearsed, its performance still represents a major achievement for the diverse community of performers, who were able to communicate successfully despite their different native languages. Cherkaoui and Jalet's metaphor of cooperation is a utopian proposition, which seems to offer hope of a possibility of overcoming the confusion of languages and cultures characterised by the Babel story. This will be developed further in the next section, by drawing particular attention the alternative of the universal language of the body, beyond the manipulation of Gormley's frames alone.

Overcoming Babel, Imperialism and Language Dominance

Following the collision between the different metallic structures, the performers begin to apologise profusely to each other, each in their own language, seeming overly keen to take the blame for the accident. This develops into a language competition, including tongue twisters in the performers' different languages. Later in the work, the other performers are clustered around Woods's body, a couple at his feet, a couple at his arms crossing their arms in front of his chest like armour, one with his legs wrapped around his waist holding his knees and one holding his hands around his head like a horned helmet, so that he resembles a Transformer figure. He speaks through a device that transforms his voice, making it sound deeper and more metallic. He tells Ducharme, one of the people who most unashamedly speaks French in the work, to 'Shut the fuck up' and advances forward with loud and destructive thuds. Unimpressed, Ducharme casually points at him and asks the audience 'Qu'est-ce que c'est, cette connerie américaine?', which translates as 'What's this American bullshit?'. This response evokes a refusal of French culture to be dominated by Anglophone influence. Ducharme inquires who on earth has made this choreography, because he is not impressed, but before he can finish his sentence, he is 'shot' down by Woods. To percussive Indian *tabla* music, the configuration of the other dancers around Woods's body becomes more elaborate. They extend his shooting arms, he launches another performer through the space like a missile and he shoots several automated guns at once. One performer cartwheels with bent arms and legs like a ninja star until she hits another performer in the chest. Woods emits deep, evil-sounding laughter. The scene brings to mind notions of US military dominance. Everyone then spins upstage and gathers behind Woods. One by one they align themselves extending their arms next to his, interlinking, until they form giant wings. These wings sequentially move up and down.

Then, Woods perches on top of the other performers as if he is sitting on a throne. Several arms stick out behind his head, fingers jutting out, like the antlers of a trophy animal on a wall. One performer is face down on the floor, arms extended, resembling a rug made out of an animal hide with the head still attached, echoing the décor of a colonial trophy room. Woods, an African American performer, sits cross-legged in a slightly effeminate manner, in an image of striking postcolonial complexity. Woods launches a celebration of English as the best language in the world, while he treads on, sits on and clobbers the other dancers. This scene was briefly discussed in Chapter 5 as part of an investigation of heteroglossia and non-translation in Cherkaoui's work, to indicate that in *Babel*^(*words*) Cherkaoui and Jalet alert spectators to the issues with translating for the dominant language's sake. He says: 'English is the most widespread language in the world and is more widely spoken and written than any other language. Over 400 million people use the English vocabulary as a mother tongue, only surpassed in numbers, but not in distribution by speakers of the many varieties of Chinese. Over 700 million people, speak English, as a foreign language. [...] English is the medium for 80% of the information stored in the world's computers. [...] No language has more synonyms than English. [The other performers have arranged themselves lying face down on the floor next to one another, with Kozuki lying across their backs. Woods sits on top of Kozuki and the others start to roll sideways, thereby carrying Woods across with them. It signifies the ultimate objectification and exploitation of the world's resources and human labour by colonial powers.] English is the language of the King of Pop, Michael Jackson, the King of Rock 'n Roll, Elvis Presley, the Queen of Pop, Madonna, the Queen of Soul, Areth Franklin, Prince and Lady Gaga. English is the language of aviation and, thank you, God, Christianity. [...] People who count English as their mother tongue make up less than 10% of the world's population, but possess over 30% of the world's economic power. Therefore, in terms of the quantity of transmitted information, English is the leader by far. Of the 163 nations of the UN, more choose English as their official language than any other. English is the language of my dear, dear friend and colleague, Queen Elizabeth II, and is the only language in which she speaks of herself in the plural: "We are not amused". English is the language of the world's greatest authors: William Shakespeare, Stephen King, and Jackie Collins. In English, we can distinguish between a house and a home, as for instance, the French cannot [Leboutte interjects saying in French that that is not true]. English is the language of the Royal Ballet. English is the language transmitted by the world's five largest television broadcasting networks: CBS, ABC, NBC, BBC and CBC, reaching millions and millions of people all around the world. English is the language of the most powerful man in the world, President Barack Hussain Obama. The Oxford English Dictionary now has twenty volumes, 615,000 entries, 2,412,000 supporting quotations and over 350 million keystrokes of text, one for every native English-speaking person in the world. Yes, English is the best language ever invented and it was the language I was born to speak. People who don't speak English are illiterate by global terms. And why would you want to speak another language anyway, because they're all so boring'. In this scene of unbelievable irony, it is inconceivable that the African American Woods would not be sensitive to the issues of power that have stemmed from colonisation, which has led to the spread of English in the British Empire. This celebration of English, acted out atop a landscape of objectified Others, is entirely oblivious to the reasons why English has become such an important language. These colonial and imperialist agendas are conveniently ignored, yet, it is precisely by their overt omission from the work that the scene becomes so hilarious and intolerable at the same time.

Ducharme gets up on his feet and emphatically says to the audience that if there is one language that has had a defining mark on poetry, theatre and love, it is French. Leboutte interjects by saying 'Ik hou van u' and 'Ich liebe dich', meaning 'I love you' in Flemish and German. The South-African Michael advances and asks 'Nederlands? And what is the most famous word in Nederlands? Apartheid'. She goes on to say that in her country, they speak eleven languages and lists them. Benaji interrupts her and begins to speak in Arabic. Woods interrupts him, saying 'Thank you, thank you, now just go back to your country'. So, it continues with Swedish, Portuguese, Italian and Japanese also making an appearance. One of the metal frames is lowered down and becomes a boxing ring, in which a contest follows by performers shouting out tongue twisters in different languages. This word-contest then escalates into a fight, albeit slow motion, resembling war action paintings by Rubens (*Massacre of the Innocents*, c. 1611) and Delacroix (*Liberty Leading the People*, c. 1830). One clambers on top of the others to seek dominance, but is immediately replaced on top of the formation by another, in an endless and random cycle of violence. Bovi and Leboutte harmonise and upturn the boxing ring, so that it becomes a picture frame for this tableau vivant. At the end, they all fall down. From the battleground, a touching duet by Chaudhari and Fournier emerges, clutching on to each other's naked torsos. Leboutte then sweeps all the lifeless bodies upstage with a broom. The musicians provide a transcultural collage of musical practices, Japanese flute layered on top of Sufi singing. Woods tentatively revisits some fragments of the texts of his earlier speeches, all muddled together and rendered nonsensical. Yet, the fragmented mise-en-scène of diverse cultural elements has by now become a very familiar aspect of Cherkaoui's aesthetic and, in this case, gives the spectator some time for reflection (Fig. 7.3).

During the summer 2009, when I observed and witnessed the initial workshop stages of the creation process, the Turkish musician Fahrettin Yarkin came to work with the dancers, which led to the creation of a key scene called 'Zikr'. I joined in with the workshops. We practised a Sufi singing exercise called *Zikr*, which means 'pronouncing Allah'.

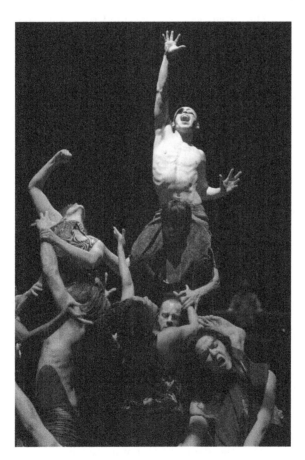

Fig. 7.3 *Babel⁽ʷᵒʳᵈˢ⁾* by Sidi Larbi Cherkaoui and Damien Jalet (Photo by Koen Broos)

He explained that the root is making rhythms with the heartbeat and breathing. No special talent is needed; you just do it and get in trance. *Zikr* is normally done in big groups, where the leader gives the main rhythm and everyone follows. It starts slowly and gradually becomes faster, then reaches its peak and slows down again. Normally people stand very close together to facilitate the transmission of energy. In January 2010, I saw Fournier create movements that corresponded to this rhythm. He was seated in fourth position on the floor, and on the inhalation, he lifted up, suspended, with his head thrown back and chest lifted up high. The exhalation corresponded to a collapsing back onto the floor. When I came back in March 2010, this movement idea had been developed into an elaborately choreographed scene. The dancers performed movements such as vigorously swinging their head in a figure of eight shape and rising from and sinking to the floor, closely corresponding to the Sufi rhythm. It seemed that the sense of gravity is heightened in their movements, but that they were constantly struggling against it. Their movements became exhausted and Cherkaoui and Jalet found—corporeally 'honest', which can be taken to mean devoid of mannerisms and individual style. This exhausting movement, focusing entirely on the rhythms of the breath, is therefore posited as one which transcends language. The three protagonists, Leboutte, Svensson and Woods look in on the scene from the side of the stage. When everyone is exhausted and stands to catch their breath, Svensson trots to the front, extends her arms wide and ushers everyone to the back of the stage.

The final scene of the work shows the dancers standing in a line next to each other facing the audience. Woods is in the middle and Svensson and Leboutte are on either side of the line. They hook one foot behind the leg of the performer next to them. Like this, they walk sequentially, one by one, the back leg pulling the next person's front leg forwards. They exaggerate the movements of the upper body in trying to keep balance. The performers use their hands to help and support the next person and pull them up. This scene shows the dancers working together, cooperating in a different way to that required for the manipulation of Gormley's aluminium structures, and Cherkaoui and Jalet find that this formation might express the idea of a common project. It is significant that the dancers are connected in this scene through touch. Although it may seem like an impediment at first to be connected at the feet, like a three-legged race but with thirteen people, the theatrical image created is very strong, not least in the simplicity of movement and the element of repetition. It works on spectators in an affective way, inviting them to imagine what it feels like to move together in this way, negotiating balance and locomotion in a large group of connected people. The choreographers chose to end the piece with a message of recovery and hope. The final image shows that the solution to the Babel problem is 'honest' movement, a surrendering to rhythm and gravity and 'common' touch. In other words, for Cherkaoui and Jalet, people from diverse cultures can be connected through dance and bodywork as a transcultural act, which they propose are an antidote to conflict and misunderstanding as a result of language confusion.

Cherkaoui and Jalet's *Babel*$^{(words)}$ was introduced as a work that brought together eighteen performers from thirteen different countries, who express themselves in fifteen different languages. The work provides a critical geopolitical evaluation of territoriality, national identity and language through choreographic exploration of several relevant themes, including borders and border controls, the Old Testament story of Babel and the perception of space as organised, delineated and transformed by Gormley's moveable cuboid aluminium frames. As part of my continuous dramaturgical engagement with the work as a spectator and scholar, this chapter has located *Babel*$^{(words)}$ within the context of the fracturing, multinational Belgian state, which is characterised by federal instability and political impasse, but also considers how Cherkaoui and Jalet move the discussion beyond the Belgian context. The manipulation and constant resignification of Gormley's cuboid frames visualise a continuous shifting of the meanings around space, territory, power and identity. Created in the wake of the global economic crisis of 2008, the work critically interrogates the workings of geopolitics, capitalism and neoliberal policies and their consequences for people of different social classes to inhabit certain spaces. Deep-seated colonial histories are brought to the fore in language battles that escalate to the acute levels of misunderstanding, characteristic of the Babel story. The possibility of hope and recovery is situated in a return to the body and is exemplified in the Sufi practice of 'Zikr', which exaggerates the breath with movement towards exhaustion in a transcendental ritual or through the simple linking of limbs as a group and uniting through touch.

BIBLIOGRAPHY

Appadurai, Arjun. *Modernity at Large: Cultural Dimensions of Globalization.* Minneapolis: University of Minnesota Press, 1996. Print.

Benjamin, Walter. *Illuminations.* New York: Schocken Books, 1968. Print.

Cherkaoui, Sidi Larbi & Jalet, Damien. *Sidi Larbi Cherkaoui onderzoekt met dansers uit vijf continenten de band tussen taal en territorium, tussen identiteit en religie. De toren van Babel.* 2010. Web. Interview. Accessed: 13 April 2010. <http://www.cobra.be/cm/cobra/podium/100408-sa-sidi_larbie_cherkaoui>.

Dodds, Klaus. *Geopolitics: A Very Short Introduction.* Oxford: Oxford University Press. 2007. Print.

Foucault, Michel. *Discipline and Punish: The Birth of the Prison.* 2nd Ed. London: Vintage Books, 1995. Print.

Krauss, Nicole. *The History of Love.* London: W. W. Norton, 2006. Print.

Olaerts, An. 'Marokkaan uit Hoboken én Choreograaf van het Jaar'. *Vacature.* 31 October 2008. 14–17. Print.

Ramachandran, Vilayanur. *The Neurons That Shaped Civilization.* 2009. Online TED Lecture. Accessed: 3 February 2010. <http://www.ted.com/talks/vs_ramachandran_the_neurons_that_shaped_civilization.html>.

Schmitz, Christoph; Domagala, Josef & Haag, Petra. *Handbook of Aluminium Recycling: Fundamentals, Mechanical Preparation, Metallurgical Processing, Plant Design.* Essen: Vulkan-Verlag, 2006. Print.

Multimedia Sources

Babel(*words*). Co-choreographed by Sidi Larbi Cherkaoui and Damien Jalet. 2010. Video Recording of Performance.

Dogville. Written and directed by Lars von Trier. 2003. Film.

The Offensive Translator. Written by Catherine Tate. 2006. Web. Accessed: 1 February 2019. <https://www.youtube.com/watch?v=XY66ZJ0TFUI>.

Interview

Seabra, Helder. Interview with author. Brussels, March 2010.

CHAPTER 8

Final Reflections

In April 2015, the National Youth Dance Company (NYDC) premiered Cherkaoui's work *Frame[d]* at Sadler's Wells in London. Since 2012, the NYDC, supported by the Department of Education and Arts Council England, offers talented young performers the opportunity to perform work led by renowned choreographers. For the 2014–15 season, Cherkaoui served as Guest Artistic Director and, for this commission, reimagined moments from his repertoire; *Babel^(words)* (co-choreographed with Damien Jalet, 2010), *Loin* (2005), *Puz/zle* (2012) and *TeZukA* (2011). *Frame[d]* is thus an amalgamated work, consisting of excerpts, which are repurposed, recontextualised and resignified by the large, young cast of 38 performers. Cherkaoui highlights that he enjoys 'a sense of transformation; I don't want things to become fixed. … It is good to look at things from different perspectives, to turn them upside down and get another view of the world – you can read the world in the work' (Cherkaoui 'Creating Frame[d]'). So, the work becomes concerned with the experience of young people finding their place in the world, among *Babel^(words)*'s metallic cuboid frames, rescaled by Antony Gormley to allow for touring to smaller venues. He brought on board key collaborators from his company Eastman to act as Assistant Choreographers, namely Navala Chaudhari, Leif Firnhaber, Elias Lazaridis and Elie Tass. These are all performers who had been part of some of those original creations.

During the creative process of *Babel^(words)*, Cherkaoui and Jalet used two pieces of electronic music by the New York electroclash performance

© The Author(s) 2019
L. Uytterhoeven, *Sidi Larbi Cherkaoui*, New World Choreographies,
https://doi.org/10.1007/978-3-030-27816-8_8

artists, Fischerspooner, to accompany the creation of the 'programming' scene and the scene based on intricate geometrical walking patterns. However, in *Babel*$^{(words)}$, in keeping with Cherkaoui's insistence on live music in his works, the rhythms of the two popular songs were recreated by the live musicians, which created an interesting transcultural aural landscape based on instruments and musical practices from Japan, India and the Mediterranean region. *Frame[d]* sees the return to the original electronic versions, probably due to budgetary reasons. As a result of this artistic decision, the original lyrics of the Fischerspooner song 'We need a war' find their way into the work and begin to interact with the drama-turgical layers in ways that did not exist in the original work:

> We need a war
> We need a war to show 'em
> We need a war to show 'em that we can
> We need a war to show 'em that we can do it
> Whenever we say we need a war.
> If they mess with us
> If we think they might mess with us
> If we say they might mess with us
> If we think we need a war, we need a war. (Fischerspooner)

The large group of dancers embark on a *mandala*-shaped walking pattern. They traverse a circle along its different axes and trace the circumference with their footsteps. The walking turns into running. Some of the dancers throw in acrobatic tricks such as cartwheels, flips and jumps. The dancers begin to collide and fall down. The scene ends with all but one of the dancers lying motionless on the peripheries of the stage, resembling the casualties of war. This theatrical image represents the human costs of state-driven warfare.

A lone figure, a young man, surveys the corpses on the battlefield, perhaps looking for his brothers or friends. He grabs hold of the wrist of one body with one hand, and then another with his other hand. He pulls and twists the bodies into a dance, animating them, infusing the puppet-like bodies with motion and life. One trio is particularly touching, a strong emotional evocation of humanity. The other bodies wriggle and migrate into two lines spanning the whole width of the stage. The bodies lie top to tail and their hands clasp their neighbour's wrist. The young man and his two puppets are in the centre and initiate waves, rippling to either side. The bodies bend at the waist, torsos collapsing over legs, and extend again. They roll backwards over their shoulders until they lie face down. The bodies wriggle again and migrate into a huge pile centre stage. Bodies are contorted, thrown haphazardly together, reminiscent of images of genocide. The lone survivor climbs to the top and looks up to the heavens for some kind of rescue, but none comes, and this image is the end of the performance.

The performances of *Frame[d]* happened in the midst of a controversy in the UK about the standards of contemporary dance training. Three choreographers, Lloyd Newson, Akram Khan and Hofesh Shechter, released a joint statement lamenting their inability to recruit high standard professional dance graduates from three leading British contemporary dance vocational colleges (BBC News *Akram Khan Criticises Quality*). While there are many complex factors underlying current issues in the state of British contemporary dance training, for example, the complex tensions between rigorous technique training and the vital principles of somatic practice and the pressures arising from its positioning within the larger marketisation of higher education, the choreographers' call for greater rigour, strength and discipline was nothing if not provocative. Cherkaoui's work with NYDC signalled that he held a somewhat different view on the issue. Dance critic Sanjoy Roy interviewed Cherkaoui for the programme booklet:

> How, I ask, does he [Cherkaoui] find dealing with not just such a large bunch but such a mixed bunch, both in terms of dance training and personal background? "I like that they have to co-exist," he replies. "My own company, Eastman, is a little like that, so in a way it's familiar to me. I like diversity. I know some people think it is dangerous in dance, that what we need is integrity and coherence. And I think: no, no! The older I get, the more convinced I am that what dance needs is diversity, different points of view. So that our creations are as informed as we can make them. That can only come from people approaching things in different ways." (Roy)

Cherkaoui's work enabled the individual personalities of the 38 dancers to shine through. *Frame[d]* does not seek out uniformity. One simple way in which Cherkaoui enables diversified expression is that all the dancers could design and put together their own costume. More crucially, one of the dancers, Annie Edwards, visibly stands out in the work due to her short appearance, as she has a growth disorder. Yet, her presence is never framed as a problem; instead, her particular identity and the dramaturgical potential that it brings with it are unleashed creatively in the work. This is not the first time Cherkaoui has worked with a disabled performer; already at the start of his career he worked with Theater Stap on *Ook* (2002), where he met Marc Wagemans and Ann Dockx, the former of whom then joined him for *Foi* (2003) and both of whom were part of the cast of *Myth* (2007). His creative process is not intent on making dancers fit in with his choreographic aesthetic; rather, he takes his collaborators' experience and humanity as the starting point for transcultural exchange, mutual learning and co-shaping of the work's dramaturgy. In contrast to the press release of the other three choreographers, the relationship Cherkaoui envisages with the performers with whom he collaborates is not simply one of employer and employee.

Instead, Cherkaoui's emphasis on dramaturgical process, diversity and co-existence as the core aim for his Guest Artistic Directorship for NYDC could translate on a wider scale. He explains:

> Throughout the process, it has been interesting to see how the elements from different works connect and speak to each other, finding a common thread that runs through the pieces to create a different story, giving new meaning in a fresh context; this also links to the idea of us all being connected. I like to sketch out the work quite vaguely, to give space for clarity to rise, trusting inspiration to come and enjoying the moment of not knowing. This allows the dancers to find their place in the piece and contribute their ideas and movement qualities. (Cherkaoui 'Creating Frame[d]')

The connection between Cherkaoui's interest in collaboration with diverse casts and the continuous dramaturgical process of resignification comes to the fore in this quote. The different chapters in this book have envisaged how this continuous process also includes the spectator.

TRANSFORMING CULTURE, NATION, RELIGION AND LANGUAGE

This book has examined the ways in which Cherkaoui questions and challenges Western, hegemonic conceptions of the nation, culture, religion and language through his work. In this final chapter, I wish to highlight the connections between the micro and macro dramaturgies of his works in this regard, as well as linking these back to the key choreographic themes and dramaturgical strategies identified through an initial analysis of his early work *Rien de Rien* (2000) in Chapter 2. These choreographic themes were:

1. gestural hand movements and choreographed storytelling
2. the citation of popular and folk dance practices
3. circular bodily movements akin to calligraphy
4. manipulation, power play and the literal objectification of dancing bodies
5. extreme virtuosity, contortionism and inversion.

and the dramaturgical strategies were:

1. the creative exploration of postcolonial and 'Other' subjectivity
2. the privileging of orally transmitted songs and stories
3. self-reflexive, dance historical references
4. heteroglossia and non-translation of foreign languages
5. choreographed iconography of a religious nature to be excavated
6. a complex mise-en-scène, characterised by simultaneity.

Many of these micro-dramaturgical strategies and choreographic approaches cluster together and intersect with one another, as well as with the larger macro-dramaturgical concerns that have emerged from Cherkaoui's oeuvre through analysis of the key selected works from the 2000–2010 period in the previous chapters:

1. political resistance to nationalism and populism
2. transculturality
3. transreligious approaches to understanding human experience
4. postcolonial problematising of translation
5. Jungian psychoanalysis
6. critical geopolitics.

However, it is impossible to neatly align these three lists; rather choreography, micro and macro dramaturgy form intricate and dynamic webs that resist being pinned down. Instead the choreographic and dramaturgic webs invite spectators to engage in a sort of play, or dance, with the fragments of incomplete meaning with which they are presented.

Chapters 2 and 7, focusing on *Rien de Rien* and *Babel*^(words) respectively, are both macro-dramaturgically concerned with the nation as construct, meaning that they somehow seek to transform populist, right-wing ways of thinking about the nation. The analysis of *Rien de Rien* is informed by an exploration of the complexity of the Belgian state, in which political power is spread amongst rainbow coalitions consisting of multiple parties within the consociational model. *Rien de Rien* is read as a disarming critique of the Flemish populist radical right made from Cherkaoui's subjectivity as an 'allochthonous' young man. With the realisation that Belgium's political complexity could in fact be seen to have tempered the spread of populist radical right ideology, the premise was set up that Cherkaoui has become drawn to staging complexity in his choreographic works as a micro-dramaturgical strategy. The complexity is achieved through foregrounding the diverse and Other subjectivities of the cast, through the fragmented storytelling, through the non-translation of foreign languages, and through the wide-ranging musical elements that form the aural landscape. This micro-dramaturgical complexity poses significant dramaturgical challenges for spectators, who are unable to easily derive linear or straightforward meanings from the work. Cherkaoui's dramaturgical collaboration with De Vuyst on *Rien de Rien* then becomes a blueprint for the further development of his approach to dramaturgy and composition in his later works and is driven to the extreme in *Myth*, the mise-en-scène of which is intensely multi-layered and characterised by simultaneity. In this sense, Cherkaoui can be seen to build on the Flemish approach to new dramaturgies, instigated by people like Marianne Van Kerkhoven, who posits that: 'Dramaturgy today is often a case of solving puzzles, learning to deal with complexity. This management of complexity demands an investment from all the senses, and, more especially, a firm trust in the path of intuition' ('Looking' 148). While Van Kerkhoven was writing about the role of the dramaturg, her call for engagement with dramaturgical complexity can be extended to the work performed by the spectator in making sense of Cherkaoui's multi-layered works.

Cherkaoui's work is intent on challenging the narrow thinking of nationalism, introduced in the Flemish political context in Chapter 1, and in destabilising the concept of the nation itself, interrogated through a focus on transculturality in Chapter 3. In Maalouf's writing on identity as composite and characterised by multiplicity, Cherkaoui found affirmation of his kaleidoscopic approach to identity as fragmented, ever-shifting and constantly realigned and reoriented. For Cherkaoui, national identity is but one aspect of identity and he is cautious of allowing it to overpower the other dimensions of identity. I have suggested that cosmopolitanism is another concept with which Cherkaoui aligns himself and his practice. He is interested in what people have in common, rather than what sets them apart, and entertains the idea that dance, rhythm and movement play a key role in that, while his utopian aim is to improve understanding between people from different cultures (Olaerts). Cosmopolitanism as a concept is based on the utopian notion that all human beings belong to the same community and have responsibilities of justice and hospitality towards each other beyond state boundaries. Cherkaoui's dance company, and by extension his choreographic work, exemplifies this kind of cosmopolitan openness to different cultures, languages, dance idioms, musicalities, approaches and ideas. He, the company, and the work itself, travel the world in a cosmopolitan way, either as part of creation or performance.

This cultural permeability of Cherkaoui's work aligns itself well with the notion of transculturality. One dimension of cosmopolitan discourse is that cultures are seen as always already mixed and hybrid, and therefore the notion of cultural purity is untenable. Cherkaoui negotiates this permeability of cultures choreographically with Khan in *zero degrees* (2005), discussed in Chapter 3. He dismantles the Hebrew song 'Jerusalem of Gold', which has grown into a symbol of militant Israeli nationalism, by unveiling the song's illegitimate Basque roots in order to reveal the nation as construct. The origin of this song and Cherkaoui's reasons underpinning his choice for including it in the work came to light in an informal conversation with Cherkaoui, which then prompted further research as part of my spectatorial dramaturgical activity. This continuous engagement with certain elements from *zero degrees* and *Babel(words)* established with confidence that Cherkaoui's choreographic negotiations of geopolitical critique and national identity were grounded in his awareness of transcultural appropriation of cultural practices and the cosmopolitan permeability of culture, and an understanding of identity as kaleidoscopic, fragmented, composite and continually shifting and realigned.

Also in Chapter 3, Cherkaoui's choreographic representations of storytelling were discussed with regard to postcolonial writings on the genre of the travel story. Theorising the travel story helps to conceive of it as being generated from 'contact zones' or 'social spaces where disparate cultures meet, clash, and grapple with each other' (Pratt 7). Beyond the eighteenth-century travel writing Pratt considers as a historian, contact zones can be a useful notion in order to make sense of travel, tourism and migration in the globalised world. It is argued that Cherkaoui actively explores and exploits contact zones, especially through working with performers who are aware of the contact zones within the Self due to migration or mixedness, as these tend to reveal cultural difference and friction. Abu-Lughod makes a case for halfie-ethnography by people whose identity is mixed, proposing to favour the writing of 'ethnographies of the particular' that focus on individual decision-making as opposed to generalisation and seemingly neutral description. Likewise, Cherkaoui's exploration of particular cultural elements, such as stories, songs and movement practices, can be read as 'choreographies of the particular', because he presents cultural difference beyond the stereotypical, challenging Western hegemony and ethnocentrism.

The stories in Cherkaoui's work are given specific choreographic treatment, for example, by duplicating the storytelling in another body in unison in *Rien de Rien* and *zero degrees*. Ripped out of their original context, these stories raise questions about who is speaking and where and when the story is set precisely. In a heightened affective engagement, the spectator flits between intently listening to the story and being distracted by the unison duplication of the story and the body language. This seems to work towards both destabilising and heightening perception. It may cause the stories and images to linger in the spectator's mind long after the performance, so that the questions raised by the stories can be engaged with as part of the continuous dramaturgy of the spectator.

For Benjamin in his 1936 essay 'The Storyteller', the oral transmission of knowledge is something pre-modern that was lost due to the mass production of the novel in modern society and needed to be mourned. Cherkaoui re-claims the value of the subjective and the orally transmitted through his celebration of storytelling in his work. He gives a platform to a wide range of alternative voices in his works, for example, the stories of victims of the atomic bomb attacks in Japan during the Second World War in *Foi* and *Myth* and can therefore be seen to challenge the elevation of the written word.

Appadurai's notion of scapes becomes an important theoretical lens through which to engage with Cherkaoui's work. Scapes can be considered as complex, flowing, overlapping building blocks that can be used to imagine the modern world, in favour of fixed landscapes. Initially, Appadurai's ethnoscapes—or the people who travel the world, which could include tourists, guest workers, immigrants and refugees—help us to understand Cherkaoui's highlighting of performers' stories that talk of displacement and cultural clashes. The inclusion of stories that are available online, via TED or YouTube, raises further questions about Appadurai's mediascapes. Mediascapes refer to the electronic production and dissemination of information through the mass, broadcast and post-broadcast media and also include the 'large and complex repertoires of images, narratives, and ethnoscapes' created by these mediascapes (Appadurai 35). In his works, Cherkaoui taps into these messy repertoires of images and stories, brought to the creation through the performers' personal experience or through exploration of online material. Like mediascapes, Cherkaoui's works also consist of image-centred, narrative-based fragments and function for the spectator in a similar way, as through the engagement with Cherkaoui's work spectators also transform it into imagined wholes. However, while Cherkaoui mimics the workings of mediascapes in his works, he also departs from these as unspoken and uncritical doings, by placing the stories told in his works under increased scrutiny through a heightened affective engagement, as discussed in relation to the continuous spectatorial dramaturgy.

In his works, Cherkaoui negotiates the forcible construction of identity through exclusionary social categories in modernity. He also highlights the role of the written word in establishing and perpetuating such social categories. It is argued that he counteracts this modernity through the inclusion of storytelling and orally transmitted songs. In contrast to Benjamin's mourning of a lost pre-modern state of being, Cherkaoui actively negotiates his own reality of transnational collaboration and intercultural exchange and can be seen to operate in a worldwide and uncontrollable 'modernity at large' (Appadurai).

The contextualisation and emerging theorisation of religious fundamentalisms demonstrated that the tensions around new totalitarianism and Islamophobia are complex and the debates ongoing. The border between freedom of speech and hate speech is one of the key arguments to be negotiated in the present by any cultural actor. In this context, Chapter 4 evaluated Cherkaoui's choreographic negotiations of the transreligious in *Foi* and *Apocrifu* (2007), given that his life has been located at the crossroads of religious tensions in Western Europe. It is argued that Cherkaoui positions himself very carefully in this complex debate. By choreographing the intertextuality of the Holy texts of Judaism, Christianity and Islam in *Apocrifu*, Cherkaoui visualises the content of a YouTube speech by Reverend Jay Smith. A selected section from this speech is later staged by Cherkaoui, precisely because Smith's argument that the texts are man-made and have been subject to editorial amendments throughout the centuries supports Cherkaoui's distrust of the literal interpretation of the religious Word within fundamentalism. However, at the same time as reiterating this specific section of Smith's online speech, it is argued that Cherkaoui also distances himself from both Smith's apparent ethnocentric agenda and the ensuing online hate speech in response to the video, which exposes the rigidities of both Christian and Muslim fundamentalisms, through humour and resignification (Butler). Cherkaoui's carefully balanced choreographic negotiation within this complex argument reveals the limitations of the Western Enlightenment worldview now that it has come under stress due to wild appropriation and mistranslation in the globalised world, as has been argued by Appadurai with ideoscapes.

In *Myth*, however, Cherkaoui finds an alternative choreographic strategy to destabilise religious fundamentalism by visualising the Jungian psychoanalytical concept of the circumambulation of symbols. Positing religion as a kind of myth, he choreographs the cross as a flexible, fluid symbol, which reveals its shifting and elusive meanings as it wanders in front of the eye of the spectator. Hence, singular meanings and reductive interpretation are discouraged. Circumambulation, a central part of Hindu and Buddhist devotional practice, becomes relevant in the signification process too, as a parallel was established between the 'walking around' symbols when excavating dreams during analysis and the dramaturgical labour on the part of the spectator, who engages with the performance retrospectively.

Chapter 5 examined examples of heteroglossia and non-translation from *Myth* in relation to postcolonial critiques of non-translation. It was explained that the heteroglossia in Cherkaoui's work is the result of cross-cultural collaborative devising processes, which are, to a certain extent, visible and audible in the staged work. Carlson's discussion of heteroglossic theatre as characterised by cultural difference, collective creation and open-endedness as a response to new multicultural audiences holds some validity with regard to Cherkaoui's work. However, I have argued that Cherkaoui's heteroglossic dramaturgy exceeds the potential of heteroglossic theatre to oppose nationalism ascribed to it by Carlson. Cherkaoui's dramaturgy of non-translation problematises, and even undermines, the signification process, as meaning appears hidden to the spectators, who are left to their own devices to 'make sense' of the performance. Even after the poststructuralist labour on behalf of the spectator of imaginative play (Adshead-Lansdale), spectators still do not understand everything in Cherkaoui's work. Likewise, Cherkaoui's practice challenges the notion of dramaturgy as mediation between artist and audience (Turner & Behrndt). However, in line with postcolonial critiques that emphasised the limitations of translation (Spivak; Venuti) extending Benjamin's argument in the 1923 essay 'The Task of the Translator', Cherkaoui's rejects the role of translator and the idea that he has an obligation to translate for the audience. His deliberate dramaturgies of non-translation give rise to the continuous dramaturgical engagement of the spectator, as he invites the spectator to feel, appreciate, respond to and reflect on what it is like to experience the jarring need for translation and to be between cultures, histories and identities. The labour that he invites spectators to engage in may entail cross-cultural conversations with others after the performance moment.

The paradox of Cherkaoui's dramaturgies lies in the fact that he translates, guides and explains less, in order for spectators to begin to understand more through their own continuous dramaturgical work. In this way, he may be getting closer to achieving his utopian aim of improving the understanding between people of different cultures through his choreography (Olaerts). This endeavour was recognised by UNESCO in April 2011, when Cherkaoui was honoured for promoting dialogue across cultures.

A key aspect of dramaturgically engaged spectatorship is the result of the visual and affective impact of Cherkaoui's choreography. Both the corporeal, in terms of how Cherkaoui choreographs the movements of the body with a focus on sometimes extreme virtuosity, and the wider mise-en-scène are of significance here. On the one hand, Cherkaoui's choreography emphasises bodies that are manipulated by other performers or by imagined external forces, resulting in risky images of the body being thrashed violently through space. Spectators tend to be unsettled by these kinds of movements and bodies on edge, imbued with danger and pain. On the other hand, there is a preference for rounded, circular and continuous movement—movement that never stops—which can be seen to be influenced by Arabic calligraphy and architecture, and Eastern philosophy and bodily practices, such as yoga and some martial arts.

These movements counteract the discomforting effects on spectators of the violently manipulated body by eliciting affect as they draw spectators into an endless cycle of soft, smooth and refined choreography. These sections of choreography have a resonance with scenes from *Babel*$^{(words)}$ and *Myth*, in which objects—respectively the metallic frames designed by Antony Gormley and a set of two wooden poles—are manipulated in various ways so that different images wander in front of the eye of the spectator and multiple meanings emerge. These scenes were described to illustrate the choreographic and analytical strategy of circumambulation. With Cherkaoui's corporeal exploration of roundedness and continuous choreography, the 'object' that is circumambulated is the body itself.

In terms of the wider mise-en-scène of Cherkaoui's choreography, a preference for visual complexity and simultaneity can be discerned, especially in his works for larger groups of performers as opposed to his duets. Multiple actions happen at the same time, often at the edges of the stage, giving the choreography a centrifugal quality. Choreographic actions elude the centre of the stage, and in response the multiplicity of simultaneous actions, the spectator is forced, or perhaps invited, to make individual decisions about what to focus on. This kind of decentred choreography is not unique, but where Cherkaoui's mise-en-scène differs from the choreography by Merce Cunningham, for example, is that his choreography resembles the late medieval Flemish painting by Hieronymus Bosch and Pieter Bruegel the Elder. These paintings display multiple narrative scenes all at once, scattered all over the painting. The viewer cannot possibly take in the painting as a whole and is invited to create their own pathway through the painting, scrutinising the sometimes grotesque scenes one by one, thereby introducing the temporal dimension to taking in the painting. Cherkaoui's decentred aesthetic, like Cunningham's, can be read as a political act against the conventions of the theatre. Whereas Cunningham may be seen to denounce his authorial responsibilities as a choreographer through a reliance on chance procedures with a complete disregard for the audiences' expectations, Cherkaoui likewise challenges spectators who enter the auditorium expecting to be passively taken on a journey by the choreographer. Spectators of Cherkaoui's dance theatre are invited to be active and selective, and no one spectator will see the same elements of the performance as another. The late medieval Flemish painting to which Cherkaoui's work bears resemblance preceded the Renaissance, during which techniques of perspective were introduced. Perspective assumes an ideal vantage point, an ideal position from which the painting can be viewed in order for the perspective to work at its best. Likewise, Cherkaoui's choreography eludes the centre; seats in the centre of the auditorium are not necessarily the best places from which to watch Cherkaoui' work. However, it could also be argued that, through Cherkaoui's inclusion of elements from different cultures and his emphasis on heteroglossia and non-translation, culturally, there is no ideal vantage point from which to engage with Cherkaoui's dance theatre. The spectator is constantly invited to question his or her cultural knowledge and positioning, and the Western bias is thoroughly destabilised as adequate for the purpose of understanding Cherkaoui's work.

Dramaturgically Engaged Spectatorship

Chapter 2 outlined and discussed the discourses on new dramaturgies as they emerged in Flanders in the 1980s and 1990s and were then expanded into the Anglophone world. The main findings were that the discourses tended to be preoccupied with articulating the role of the dramaturg within the creative process. There was much less interest in exploring the relationship and interplay between the work and the spectator, although this analytical dimension is generally considered to form part of dramaturgy's twofold function (Van Kerkhoven qtd. in Turner & Behrndt).

Critical of this project of legitimation and assertion on behalf of the professional dance dramaturg, female Flemish dramaturgs De Vuyst and Van Imschoot began to raise concerns and vocalise anxieties about the perceived imbalanced power relationship between the choreographer and the dramaturg. The dramaturg seemed to embody a shortcoming in these collaborative settings, aiming to compensate for a perceived lack of capability and knowledge within the dance artist, particularly where this was an 'allochthonous' young person. Alternative dramaturgical models were considered, such as the dramaturgical context, whereby the dramaturgical responsibility was shared by a range of collaborators, including the performers. Cherkaoui's dramaturgical practice aligns itself perfectly with this approach, as—regardless of whether a professional dramaturg is employed—the whole range of artistic collaborators helps to carry this shared dramaturgical responsibility.

As a spectator, too, I have engaged in depth with the works' dramaturgies and played a role in shaping them through my own agile and ever-shifting acts of interpretation. In this context, I propose that the research method of engaged spectatorship I devised, combining observation, conversation, research and writing, is understood as a continuous dramaturgy of the spectator. In contrast to the prevailing discursive emphasis on the role of the dramaturg in the creative process, I have argued that dramaturgy continues beyond the moment of the performance on the part of the spectator, in the form of continuous dramaturgical engagement with the work's content, its imagery and religious symbolism, its aural landscape and musicological histories, its stories, its political context and poignant moments.

This book exemplifies the shapes that this continuous dramaturgical activity and engaged spectatorship may take in relation to Cherkaoui's body of work. In line with poststructural and intertextual approaches to performance analysis (e.g. Adshead-Lansdale), this increased emphasis on the role of the spectator in the dramaturgical process implies that the spectator plays a key role in the production of meaning. The artist as author is not solely in charge of signification in the performance. Cherkaoui as a choreographer, through his multi-layered works, actively seeks to open up the possibility of multiple meanings, thereby almost leaving the spectator no choice but to become active and emancipated, as proposed by Rancière. However, the most significant aspect of my argument is that this engaged spectatorship and continuous dramaturgy are needed in order for theatre to fulfil its potential for social change, as proposed in the concept of 'macro dramaturgy' (Van Kerkhoven 'Grote Dramaturgie' 69) and an 'expanded dramaturgical practice' (Eckersall 285). In this sense, theatre's potential to effectuate social change and challenge cultural norms may then begin to lead to a transformation of socio-cultural attitudes, one spectator at a time.

Engaged spectatorship hence requires an ability to analyse choreography and related micro-dramaturgical structures in the moment and articulate insights of macro-dramaturgical relevance through conversations with others and through research and writing after watching the performance. Discursive exchanges with others help spectators to remember aspect of the performance, compare experiences of the work and share in others' perspectives on the cultural aspects of the work. Engaged spectatorship is a skill that must be developed and practised, like the agility developed through dance practice itself.

It increasingly becomes possible to see a connection between the micro-dramaturgical strategies identified in Cherkaoui's work, aimed at complicating signification and drawing the spectator into a deeper hermeneutic, interpretive labour, and the macro-dramaturgical concerns that emerge from this analysis of his oeuvre, such as critical geopolitics, transreligious theology, psychoanalytical dream and symbol analysis, and musicological history. These interpretive endeavours, scholarly or otherwise, are all intent on making meaning from complex webs of materials of various natures. Critical geopolitics is concerned with understanding the political geography and international relations that characterise the globalised world. Transreligious theology seeks to comprehend how issues that are central to the human experience are approached in various religious traditions and how these overlap and inform each other, intent on undermining religious fundamentalisms. Jungian psychoanalysis focuses on the excavation of the human psyche through circumambulating the symbols that are revealed in dreams, for example, an endeavour to which the interpreter should bring 'imaginative flair' (Stevens 94).

The philosophical scholar Crysostomos Mantzavinos, in conceptualising hermeneutics, proposes that 'interpretation is a ubiquitous activity, unfolding whenever humans aspire to grasp whatever *interpretanda* they deem significant'. Juxtaposed with Van Kerkhoven's emphasis that dramaturgy is a case of learning to deal with complexity, the permeating of hermeneutic approaches into areas other than the study of the written text becomes a useful parallel that should be extended to the engaged spectatorship with dance theatre works such as Cherkaoui's. Like the transcultural conception of culture as porous and the transreligious focus on the permeability of theologies, Cherkaoui's works are porous, too, open to continuous transformation and development as spectators interact with them in a dramaturgically engaged way.

BIBLIOGRAPHY

Abu-Lughod, Lila. 'Writing Against Culture'. 1991. *Anthropology in Theory: Issues in Epistemology*. Ed. Moore, Henrietta L. & Sanders, Todd. Malden, MA: Blackwell, 2005. 466–479. Print.

Adshead-Lansdale, Janet. Ed. *Dancing Texts: Intertextuality in Interpretation*. London: Dance Books, 1999. Print.

Appadurai, Arjun. *Modernity at Large: Cultural Dimensions of Globalization*. Minneapolis: University of Minnesota Press, 1996. Print.

BBC News. 'Akram Khan Criticises Quality of UK Dance Training'. 2015. Web. Accessed: 15 July 2017. <http://www.bbc.co.uk/news/entertainment-arts-32236406>.

Benjamin, Walter. *Illuminations.* New York: Schocken Books, 1968. Print.

————. (trans. Harry Zohn) 'The Task of the Translator: An Introduction to the Translation of Baudelaire's *Tableaus Parisiens*'. *Translation Studies Reader.* Ed. Venuti, Lawrence. Florence, NY: Routledge, 1999,15–25. Print.

Butler, Judith. *Excitable Speech: A Politics of the Performative.* London: Routledge, 1997. Print.

Carlson, Marvin. *Speaking in Tongues: Language at Play in the Theatre.* Ann Arbor: The University of Michigan Press, 2006. Print.

Cherkaoui, Sidi Larbi. *Creating Frame[d].* London: Sadler's Wells, 2015. Programme Booklet.

De Vuyst, Hildegard. 'Een Dramaturgie Van Het Gebrek: Paradoxen en Dubbelzinnigheden'. *Etcetera.* 17.68. (1999): 65–66. Print.

Eckersall, Peter. 'Towards an Expanded Dramaturgical Practice: A Report on "The Dramaturgy and Cultural Intervention Project"'. *Theatre Research International.* 31.3. (2006): 283–297. Print.

Maalouf, Amin. *In the Name of Identity: Violence and the Need to Belong.* New York: Random House, 2000. Print.

Mantzavinos, Chrysostomos. 'Hermeneutics'. *Stanford Encyclopedia of Philosophy.* 2016. Web. Accessed: 1 February 2019. <https://plato.stanford.edu/entries/hermeneutics/>.

Olaerts, An. 'Marokkaan uit Hoboken én Choreograaf van het Jaar'. *Vacature.* 31 October 2008. 14–17. Print.

Pratt, Marie Louise. *Imperial Eyes: Travel Writing and Transculturation.* 2nd Ed. London: Routledge, 2007. Print.

Roy, Sanjoy. *Framing Frame[d].* London: Sadler's Wells, 2015. Programme Booklet.

Smith, Jay. 'Is the Qur'an the Word of God?'. London: Hyde Park Christian Fellowship. 1996. Web. Accessed: 18 August 2010. <http://debate.org.uk/topics/history/debate/debate.html>.

Spivak, Gayatri Chakravorty. *Outside in the Teaching Machine.* London: Routledge, 1993. Print.

Stevens, Anthony. *Jung.* Oxford: Oxford University Press, 1994. Print.

Turner, Cathy & Behrndt, Synne. *Dramaturgy and Performance.* Basingstoke: Palgrave Macmillan, 2008. Print.

Van Imschoot, Myriam. 'Anxious Dramaturgy'. *Women & Performance: A Journal of Feminist Theory.* 26.13:2. (2003): 57–68. Print.

Van Kerkhoven, Marianne. 'Looking Without Pencil in the Hand'. *Theaterschrift.* 5–6. (1994): 140–148. Print.

————. 'Van de Kleine en Grote Dramaturgie: Pleidooi voor een "Interlocuteur"'. *Etcetera.* 17.68. (1999): 67–69. Print.

————.'European Dramaturgy in the 21st Century'. *Performance Research.* 14.3. (2009): 7–11. Print.

Venuti, Lawrence. Ed. *Translation Studies Reader*. Florence, KY: Routledge, 1999. Print.

Venuti, Lawrence. *The Translator's Invisibility: A History of Translation*. 2nd Ed. London: Routledge, 2008. Print.

Multimedia Sources

Apocrifu. Choreographed by Sidi Larbi Cherkaoui. 2007. Video Recording of Performance.

Babel^(words). Co-choreographed by Sidi Larbi Cherkaoui and Damien Jalet. 2010. Video Recording of Performance.

Foi. Choreographed by Sidi Larbi Cherkaoui. 2003. Video Recording of Performance.

Is the Qur'an Corrupted?: Biblical Characters in the Qur'an. 2006. Web. Accessed: 17 August 2010. <http://www.youtube.com/watch?v=raw-SB7AjMo>.

Myth. Choreographed by Sidi Larbi Cherkaoui. 2007. Video Recording of Performance.

Rien de Rien. Choreographed by Sidi Larbi Cherkaoui. 2000. Video Recording of Performance.

Sutra. Choreographed by Sidi Larbi Cherkaoui. Sadler's Wells. Axiom Films. 2008. DVD.

'We Need a War'. Written and Performed by Fischerspooner. Odyssey. 2005. Song.

BIBLIOGRAPHY

Abu-Lughod, Lila. 'Writing Against Culture'. 1991. *Anthropology in Theory: Issues in Epistemology.* Ed. Moore, Henrietta L. & Sanders, Todd. Malden, MA: Blackwell, 2005. 466–479. Print.

Adshead, Janet. *Dance Analysis: Theory and Practice.* London: Dance Books, 1988. Print.

Adshead-Lansdale, Janet. Ed. *Dancing Texts: Intertextuality in Interpretation.* London: Dance Books, 1999. Print.

Ahmad, Dohra. '"This Fundo Stuff Is Really Something New": Fundamentalism and Hybridity in The Moor's Last Sigh'. *The Yale Journal of Criticism.* 18.1. (2005): 1–20. Print.

Appadurai, Arjun. *Modernity at Large: Cultural Dimensions of Globalization.* Minneapolis: University of Minnesota Press, 1996. Print.

Appiah, Kwame Anthony. *Cosmopolitanism: Ethics in a World of Strangers.* New York: W. W. Norton, 2006. Print.

Arfara, Katia. Aspects of a New Dramaturgy of the Spectator. *Performance Research.* 14.3. (2009): 112–118. Print.

Barba, Eugenio. *On Directing and Dramaturgy: Burning the House.* Oxon: Routledge, 2009. Print.

Bassnett, Susan & Lefevere, André. *Translation, History, and Culture.* London and New York: Pinter Publishers, 1990. Print.

Bassnett, Susan & Trivedi, Harish. *Postcolonial Translation: Theory and Practice.* London: Routledge, 1999. Print.

BBC News. 'Full Text: Writers' Statement on Cartoons'. 2006. Web. Accessed: 6 July 2012. <http://news.bbc.co.uk/1/hi/world/europe/4764730.stm>.
———. 'Akram Khan Criticises Quality of UK Dance Training'. 2015. Web. Accessed: 15 July 2017. <http://www.bbc.co.uk/news/entertainment-arts-32236406>.
Benjamin, Walter. *Illuminations*. New York: Schocken Books, 1968. Print.
———. (trans. Harry Zohn) 'The Task of the Translator: An Introduction to the Translation of Baudelaire's *Tableaux Parisiens*'. 1999. *Translation Studies Reader*. Ed. Venuti, Lawrence. Florence, NY: Routledge, 1999. 15–25. Print.
Berman, Antoine. *The Experience of the Foreign: Culture and Translation in Romantic Germany*. Albany: State University of New York Press, 1992. Print.
Bhabha, Homi K. 'Culture's In-Between'. *Questions of Cultural Identity*. Ed. Gay, Paul de & Hall, Stuart. London: Sage, 1996. 53–60. Print.
Bond, Lucy & Rapson, Jessica. Eds. *The Transcultural Turn: Interrogating Memory Between and Beyond Borders*. Berlin: Walter de Gruyter, 2014. Print.
Bossuyt, Reinout & De Lobel, Peter. 'Maak uw Eigen Coalitie'. *De Standaard Online*. 2011. Web. Accessed: 2 August 2011. <http://www.standaard.be/extra/verkiezingen/2010/coalitiekiezer>.
Bousetta, Hassan & Jacobs, Dirk. 'Multiculturalism, Citizenship and Islam in Problematic Encounters in Belgium'. *Multiculturalism, Muslims and Citizenship: A European Approach*. Ed. Modood, Tariq et al. Oxon: Routledge, 2006. 23–36. Print.
Brah, Avtar. *Cartographies of Diaspora: Contesting Identities*. Gender, Racism, Ethnicity Series. Oxon and New York: Routledge, 1996. Print.
Brizzell, Cindy & Lepecki, André. 'Introduction: The Labor of the Question Is the (Feminist) Question of Dramaturgy'. *Women & Performance: A Journal of Feminist Theory*. 26.13:2. (2003): 15–16. Print.
Butler, Judith. *Gender Trouble: Feminism and the Subversion of Identity*. London: Routledge, 1990. Print.
———. 'Performative Acts and Gender Constitution: An Essay in Phenomenology and Feminist Theory'. *Theatre Journal*. 40.4. (1990): 519–531. Print.
———. *Excitable Speech: A Politics of the Performative*. London: Routledge, 1997. Print.
Camerata Trajectina. 'Gherardus Mes - Ick seg adieu (Souterliedeken 65) (by Camerata Trajectina)'. 2010. Web. Accessed: 16 August 2018. <https://www.youtube.com/watch?v=RHeejbPHFQs>.
Capilla Flamenca – Les Ballets C. de la B. *Foi: Ars Nova, Oral Traditional Music & More*. Leuven: Capilla Flamenca, 2003. Booklet with CD.
Carlson, Marvin. *Speaking in Tongues: Language at Play in the Theatre*. Ann Arbor: The University of Michigan Press, 2006. Print.
Cherkaoui, Sidi Larbi. *Curriculum Vitae*. 1999. Unpublished Manuscript.

———. 'Eén achternaam, veel toekomst'. *MO Magazine*. 2014. Web. Accessed: 13 August 2017. <http://www.mo.be/artikel/een-achternaam-veel-toekomst>.

———. *Creating Frame[d]*. London: Sadler's Wells, 2015. Programme Booklet.

Cherkaoui, Sidi Larbi & Delmas, Gilles. *Zon-Mai: Parcours Nomades*. Arles: Actes Sud, 2007. Print.

Cherkaoui, Sidi Larbi & Jalet, Damien. *Sidi Larbi Cherkaoui onderzoekt met dansers uit vijf continenten de band tussen taal en territorium, tussen identiteit en religie. De toren van Babel*. 2010. Web. Interview. Accessed: 13 April 2010. <http://www.cobra.be/cm/cobra/podium/100408-sa-sidi_larbie_cherkaoui>.

Clair, Robin Patric. 'The Changing Story of Ethnography'. *Expressions of Ethnography: Novel Approaches to Qualitative Methods*. Ed. Clair, Robin Patric. 2003. Web. Accessed: 9 August 2018. <https://www.sunypress.edu/pdf/60804.pdf>.

Clifford, James. 'Diasporas'. *Cultural Anthropology*. 9.3. (1994): 302–338. Print.

Clifford, James & Marcus, George E. *Writing Culture: The Poetics and Politics of Ethnography*. Berkeley, CA: University of California Press, 1986. Print.

Contemporary Theatre Review. Issue on 'New Dramaturgies'. Turner, Cathy & Behrndt, Synne. Eds. 20:2. (2010). Print.

Cools, Guy. *Body: Language #1. The Mythic Body: Guy Cools with Sidi Larbi Cherkaoui*. London: Sadler's Wells, 2012. Print.

———. *In-Between Dance Cultures: On the Migratory Artistic Identity of Sidi Larbi Cherkaoui and Akram Khan*. Antennae Series. Amsterdam: Valiz, 2015. Print.

Cope, Lou. 'Sidi Larbi Cherkaoui: Myth (2007)—Mapping the Multiple'. 2010. *Making Contemporary Theatre: International Rehearsal Processes*. Ed. Harvie, Jen & Lavender, Andy. Manchester: Manchester University Press, 2010. 39–58. Print.

Coward, Harold. *Jung and Eastern Thought*. Albany: State University of New York Press, 1995. Print.

Cvejić, Bojana. 'The Ignorant Dramaturg'. *Maska*. 16.131–132. (2010): 40–53. Print.

deLahunta, Scott. 'Dance Dramaturgy: Speculations and Reflections'. *Dance Theatre Journal*. 16.1. (2000): 20–25. Print.

deLahunta, Scott; Ginot, Isabelle; Lepecki, André; Rethorst, Susan; Theodores, Diana; Van Imschoot, Myriam & Williams, David. 'Conversations on Choreography'. *Performance Research*. 8.4. (2003): 61–70. Print.

Derrida, Jacques. (trans. Samuel Weber & Jeffrey Mehlman). *Limited, Inc.* Evanston, IL: Northwestern University Press, 1988. Print.

Deschouwer, Kris. 'And the Peace Goes On? Consociational Democracy and Belgian Politics in the Twenty-First Century'. *West European Politics*. 29.5. (2006): 895–911. Print.

De Laet, Timmy. 'Giving Sense to the Past: Historical D(ist)ance and the Chiasmatic Interlacing of Affect and Knowledge'. *The Oxford Handbook of Dance and Reenactment*. Ed. Franko, Mark. Oxford: Oxford University Press, 2017. 33–56. Print.

De Standaard. 'Fotospecial: De crisis gezien door kinderogen'. 2011. Web. Accessed: 15 June 2011. <http://www.standaard.be/artikel/detail.aspx?artikelid=DMF20110611_024>.

De Vuyst, Hildegard. 'Een Dramaturgie Van Het Gebrek: Paradoxen en Dubbelzinnigheden'. *Etcetera*. 17.68. (1999): 65–66. Print.

Díaz Noci, Javier. 'The Creation of the Basque Identity Through Cultural Symbols in Modern Times'. *Ehu.es*. 1999. Web. Accessed: 20 September 2009. <http://www.ehu.es/diaz-noci/Conf/C17.pdf>.

Dobson, Nichola; Honess Roe, Annabelle; Ratell, Amy & Ruddell, Caroline. Eds. *The Animation Studies Reader*. London: Bloomsbury Academic, 2018. Print.

Dodds, Klaus. *Geopolitics: A Very Short Introduction*. Oxford: Oxford University Press, 2007. Print.

Doran, Meredith. 'Negotiating Between *Bourge* and *Racaille*: Verlan as Youth Identity Practice in Suburban Paris'. *Negotiation of Identities in Multilingual Contexts*. Ed. Pavlenko, Anna & Blackledge, Adrian. Clevedon: Multilingual Matters, 2004. 93–124. Print.

Dudek, Sarah. 'Walter Benjamin & the Religion of Translation'. *Cipher Journal*. Web. Accessed: 29 March 2011. <http://www.cipherjournal.com/html/dudek_benjamin.html>.

Duguid, Hannah. 'A Box of Delights: Antony Gormley's "Sutra"'. *The Independent*. 2008. Web. Accessed: 25 July 2018. <https://www.independent.co.uk/arts-entertainment/art/features/a-box-of-delights-antony-gormleys-sutra-831379.html>.

Eastman. 'Project/Best Belgian Dancesolo'. 2018. Web. Accessed: 24 August 2018. <http://www.east-man.be/en/14/56/>.

Eckersall, Peter. 'Towards an Expanded Dramaturgical Practice: A Report on 'The Dramaturgy and Cultural Intervention Project'. *Theatre Research International*. 31.3. (2006): 283–297. Print.

Faber, Roland. 'Der Transreligiöse Diskurs. Zu Einer Theologie Transformativer Prozesse'. *Polylog*. 9. (2002): 65–94. Print.

Faszer-McMahon, Debra. *Cultural Encounters in Contemporary Spain: The Poetry of Clara Janés*. Lewisburg, PA: Bucknell University Press. 2010. Print.

Fensham, Rachel & Kelada, Odette. 'Dancing the Transcultural Across the South'. *Journal of Intercultural Studies*. 33.4. (2012): 363–373. Print.

Flanders, Judith. 'Zero Degrees Is a True Meeting of Equals'. *Guardian Unlimited*. 2007. Web. Accessed: 9 November 2007. <http://blogs.guardian.co.uk/theatre/2007/10/zero_degrees_is_a_true_meeting.html>.

Foster, Susan L. *Reading Dancing: Bodies and Subjects in Contemporary American Dance*. Berkeley: University of California Press, 1986. Print.

Foucault, Michel. *Discipline and Punish: The Birth of the Prison*. 2nd Ed. London: Vintage Books, 1995. Print.

Franits, Wayne. *Dutch Seventeenth-Century Genre Painting*. New Haven, CT: Yale University Press, 2004. Print.

George, Rosemary Marangoly. *The Politics of Home: Postcolonial Relocations and Twentieth-Century Fiction*. Berkeley: University of California Press, 1999. Print.

Gilbert, Jenny. 'Dunas, Sadler's Wells, London: The Odd Couple Do a Sand Dance'. *The Independent*. 2011. Web. Accessed: 6 August 2018. <https://www.independent.co.uk/arts-entertainment/theatre-dance/reviews/dunas-sadlers-wells-london-2280716.html>.

Gilroy, Paul. *The Black Atlantic: Modernity and Double Consciousness*. London: Verso, 1993. Print.

Gregg, Melissa & Seigworth, Gregory J. Eds. *The Affect Theory Reader*. Durham, NC: Duke University Press, 2010. Print.

Hansen, Pil & Callison, Darcey. *Dance Dramaturgy: Modes of Agency, Awareness and Engagement*. New World Choreographies Series. London: Palgrave Macmillan, 2015. Print.

Hervé. 'Sidi Larbi Cherkaoui sur le Pont'. *Têtu*. July/August 2004.

Hyde Park Christian Fellowship. *Purpose Statement*. 1997. Web. Accessed: 18 August 2010. <http://www.debate.org.uk/info/home.htm#purpose>.

Jackson, Merilyn. 'Review: Zon-Mai'. *Philly Stage*. 2011. Web. Accessed: 19 August 2017. <http://www.philly.com/philly/blogs/phillystage/Review-Zon-Mai.html#fBYZ8qWsM4OzoYD6.99>.

Jennings, Luke. 'Dunas; May—Review'. *The Guardian*. 2011. Web. Accessed: 4 August 2018. <https://www.theguardian.com/stage/2011/may/08/dunas-sadlers-wells-review>.

Jones, Jonathan. 'Hieronymus Bosch Review—A Heavenly Host of Delights on the Way to Hell'. *The Guardian*. 2016. Web. Accessed: 30 August 2017. <https://www.theguardian.com/artanddesign/2016/feb/11/hieronymus-bosch-review-a-heavenly-host-of-delights-on-the-road-to-hell>.

Jung, Carl Gustav. (trans. R.F.C. Hull) *The Structure and Dynamics of the Psyche*. London: Routledge and Kegan Paul, 1960. Print.

———. (ed. Aniela Jaffé; trans. Richard and Clara Winston) *Memories, Dreams, Reflections*. London and Glasgow: Random House, 1963. Print.

———. (trans. R.F.C. Hull) *The Symbolic Life: Miscellaneous Writings*. London: Routledge and Kegan Paul, 1977. Print.

———. (ed. William McGuire) *Dream Analysis: Notes of the Seminar Given in 1928–1930*. London: Routledge and Kegan Paul, 1984. Print.

Kealiinohomoku, Joann. 'An Anthropologist Looks at Ballet as a Form of Ethnic Dance'. *What is Dance? Readings in Theory and Criticism*. Ed. Copeland, Roger & Cohen, Marshall. Oxford: Oxford University Press, 1983. 533–549. Print.

Khoury, Krystel. 'Un arbre aux possibilités multiples: Le traitement de la main dans le travail chorégraphique de Sidi Larbi Cherkaoui'. *Des mains modernes: Cinéma, danse, photographie, théâtre.* Ed. André, Emmanuelle; Claudia, Palazzolo & Emmanuel, Siety. Paris: L'Harmattan, 2008. 14–26. Print.

Koester, Helmut. 'Apocryphal and Canonical Gospels'. *The Harvard Theological Review.* 73.1/2. (1980): 105–130. Print.

Krauss, Nicole. *The History of Love.* London: W. W. Norton, 2006. Print.

Kudo, Satoshi. Original Japanese text cited in *Myth,* translated by Kudo, Antwerp, May 2009.

Laermans, Rudi & Gielen, Pascal. 'Flanders—Constructing Identities: The Case of 'the Flemish Dance Wave'. *Europe Dancing: Perspectives on Theatre Dance and Cultural Identity.* Ed. Grau, Andrée & Jordan, Stephanie. London: Routledge, 2000. 12–27. Print.

Lefkowitz, Natalie. *Talking Backwards, Looking Forwards: The French Language Game Verlan.* Tuebingen: Gunter Narr Verlag, 1991. Print.

Lehmann, Hans-Thies. (trans. Karen Juers-Munby) *Postdramatic Theatre.* London: Routledge, 2006. Print.

Londondance. 'Interview : Sidi Larbi Cherkaoui Q&A'. 2008. Web. Accessed: 25 July 2018. <http://londondance.com/articles/interviews/sidi-larbi-cherkaoui-qanda/>.

Lyotard, Jean-François. 'The Unconscious as Mise-en-Scène'. *Mimesis, Masochism, & Mime: The Politics of Theatricality in Contemporary French Thought.* Ed. Murray, Tim. Ann Arbor: University of Michigan Press, 1997. 163–174. Print.

Maalouf, Amin. *In the Name of Identity: Violence and the Need to Belong.* New York: Random House, 2000. Print.

Mackrell, Judith. 'Sutra'. *The Guardian.* 2008. Web. Accessed: 25 July 2018. <https://www.theguardian.com/stage/2008/may/30/dance>.

Mantzavinos, Chrysostomos. 'Hermeneutics'. *Stanford Encyclopedia of Philosophy.* 2016. Web. Accessed: 1 February 2019. <https://plato.stanford.edu/entries/hermeneutics/>.

Masalha, Nur. *The Bible and Zionism: Invented Traditions, Archaeology and Postcolonialism in Palestine-Israel.* London: Zed Books, 2007. Print.

Micrologus. *Myth—Sidi Larbi Cherkaoui: The Music.* 2007. Booklet with CD.

Miller, Henry. *The Wisdom of the Heart.* New York: New Directions Publishing, 1941. Print.

Mitra, Royona. *Akram Khan: Dancing New Interculturalism.* New World Choreographies Series. London: Palgrave Macmillan, 2015. Print.

Mnookin, Robert & Verbeke, Alain. 'Persistent Nonviolent Conflict with No Reconciliation: The Flemish and Walloons in Belgium'. *Law and Contemporary Problems.* 72:151. (2009): 151–186. Web. Accessed: 18 July 2011. <http://www.law.duke.edu/journals/lcp>.

Morin, Justin. *Sidi Larbi Cherkaoui: Pèlerinage Sur Soi.* Arles: Actes Sud, 2006. Print.

Mudde, Cas. *The Ideology of the Extreme Right.* Manchester: Manchester University Press, 2000. Print.

———. *Populist Radical Right Parties in Europe.* Cambridge: Cambridge University Press, 2007. Print.

Murray, Tim. Ed. *Mimesis, Masochism, & Mime: The Politics of Theatricality in Contemporary French Thought.* Ann Arbor: University of Michigan Press, 1997. Print.

Olaerts, An. 'Marokkaan uit Hoboken én Choreograaf van het Jaar'. *Vacature.* 31 October 2008. 14–17. Print.

Ong, Walter. *Orality and Literacy: The Technologizing of the Word.* 2nd Ed. New York: Routledge, 2002. Print.

Pavis, Patrice. (trans. David Williams) *Analyzing Performance: Theater, Dance, and Film.* Ann Arbor: University of Michigan Press, 2003. Print.

Peeters, Patrick. 'Multinational Federations: Reflections on the Belgian Federal State'. *Multinational Federations.* Ed. Burgess, Michael & Pinder, John. Oxon: Routledge, 2007. 31–49. Print.

Performance Research. Issue 'On Dramaturgy'. Gritzner, Karoline; Primavesi, Patrick & Roms, Heike. Eds. 14:3. (2009). Print.

Perusek, David. 'Grounding Cultural Relativism'. *Anthropological Quarterly.* 80.3. (2007): 821–836. Print.

Pratt, Marie Louise. *Imperial Eyes: Travel Writing and Transculturation.* 2nd Ed. London: Routledge, 2007. Print.

Ramachandran, Vilayanur. *The Neurons That Shaped Civilization.* 2009. Online TED Lecture. Accessed: 3 February 2010. <http://www.ted.com/talks/vs_ ramachandran_the_neurons_that_shaped_civilization.html>.

Rancière. Jacques. *The Emancipated Spectator.* London: Verso, 2009. Print.

Rao, Rahul. 'Postcolonial Cosmopolitanism: Between Home and the World'. D.Phil. Thesis, Politics and International Relations, University of Oxford. 2007. Web. Accessed: 15 April 2009. <http://ora.ouls.ox.ac.uk/objects/ uuid:6eb91e22-9563-49a2-be2b-402a4edd99b5>.

Renard, Han & De Ceulaer, Joël. 'De 10 machtigste en invloedrijkste allochtone landgenoten'. *Knack.* 2014. Web. Accessed: 17 July 2017. <http://www.knack.be/nieuws/mensen/de-10-machtigste-en-invloedrijk- ste-allochtone-landgenoten/article-normal-125747.html>.

Roy, Sanjoy. *Framing Frame[d].* London: Sadler's Wells, 2015. Programme Booklet.

Rushdie, Salman. *The Satanic Verses.* London: Vintage, 1988. Print.

———. *The Moor's Last Sigh.* London: Vintage, 1997. Print.

Ruthven, Malise. *Fundamentalism: A Very Short Introduction.* Oxford: Oxford University Press, 2007. Print.

Ryan, Stephen. 'Nationalism and Ethnic Conflict'. *Issues in World Politics*. Ed. White, Brian et al. 3rd Ed. Basingstoke: Palgrave Macmillan, 2005. 137–154. Print.

Sadie, Stanley. Ed. *The New Grove Dictionary of Music and Musicians*. London: Macmillan, 2001. Print.

Samuel, Raphael & Thompson, Paul Richard. *The Myths We Live By*. London: Routledge, 1990. Print.

Scanlan, Margaret. 'Writers Among Terrorists: Don DeLillo's Mao II and the Rushdie Affair'. *Modern Fiction Studies*. 40.2. (1994): 229–252. Print.

Scheffler, Samuel. *Boundaries and Allegiances: Problems of Justice and Responsibility in Liberal Thought*. Oxford: Oxford University Press, 2001. Print.

Schmitz, Christoph; Domagala, Josef & Haag, Petra. *Handbook of Aluminium Recycling: Fundamentals, Mechanical Preparation, Metallurgical Processing, Plant Design*. Essen: Vulkan-Verlag, 2006. Print.

Segev, Tom. 'Naomi Shemer Lifted Jerusalem of Gold Melody from Basque Folk Song'. *Haaretz*. 2005. Web. Accessed: 19 October 2008. <http://www.haaretz.com/naomi-shemer-lifted-jerusalem-of-gold-melody-from-basque-folk-song-1.157828>.

Seymour, Michel. *The Fate of the Nation State*. Montreal: McGill-Queen's University Press, 2004. Print.

Shryock, Andrew. *Islamophobia/Islamophilia: Beyond the Politics of Enemy and Friend*. Bloomington: Indiana University Press, 2010. Print.

Smith, Jay. 'Is the Qur'an the Word of God?' London: Hyde Park Christian Fellowship. 1996. Web. Accessed: 18 August 2010. <http://debate.org.uk/topics/history/debate/debate.html>.

Sonenberg, Janet. *Dreamwork for Actors*. London: Routledge, 2003. Print.

Sörgel, Sabine. *Dance and the Body in Western Theatre: 1948 to the Present*. London: Red Globe Press, 2015. Print.

Spivak, Gayatri Chakravorty. *Outside in the Teaching Machine*. London: Routledge, 1993. Print.

Stevens, Anthony. *Jung*. Oxford: Oxford University Press, 1994. Print.

Stevens, Mary. 'Le CNHI on Tour: la Zon-Mai and the Visual Identity'. 2007. Web. Accessed: 17 August 2017. <http://marysresearchblog.wordpress.com/2007/03/21/the-cnhi-on-tour-la-zon-mai-and-the-visual-identity/>.

Sturtewagen, Bart. 'Weg uit Logica van Winaars en Verliezers'. *De Standaard*, July 2011. Print.

Thatamanil, John J. 'Transreligious Theology as the Quest for Interreligious Wisdom: Defining, Defending, and Teaching Transreligious Theology'. *Open Theology*. 2 (2016): 354–362. Web. Accessed: 15 July 2018. <https://www.degruyter.com/downloadpdf/j/opth.2016.2.issue-1/opth-2016-0029/opth-2016-0029.pdf>.

Tierney, Stephen. *Accommodating Cultural Diversity.* Farnham: Ashgate, 2007. Print.

Turner, Cathy & Behrndt, Synne. *Dramaturgy and Performance.* Basingstoke: Palgrave Macmillan, 2008. Print.

Turner, Jane. *Eugenio Barba.* Routledge Performance Practitioners Series. Oxon: Routledge, 2004. Print.

Tutek, Hrovje. 'Limits to Transculturality: A Book Review Article of New Work by Kimmich and Schahadat and Juvan'. *CLCWeb: Comparative Literature and Culture.* 15.5. (2013). Web. Accessed: 18 August 2017. <http://docs.lib. purdue.edu/cgi/viewcontent.cgi?article=2352&context=clcweb>.

Uytterhoeven, Lise. 'Dreams, Myth, History: Sidi Larbi Cherkaoui's Dramaturgies'. *Contemporary Theatre Review.* 21.3. (2011): 332–339. Print.

Van Heuven, Robbert. 'De Dramaturg #2: Marianne Van Kerkhoven: 'Dramaturgie is de bezielde structuur van de voorstelling'. *TM: Tijdschrift over Theater, Muziek en Dans.* 9.8. (2005). 16–18. Print.

Van Imschoot, Myriam. 'Anxious Dramaturgy'. *Women & Performance: A Journal of Feminist Theory.* 26.13:2. (2003): 57–68. Print.

Van Kerkhoven, Marianne. 'Looking Without Pencil in the Hand'. *Theaterschrift.* 5.6. (1994). 140–148. Print.

———. 'Van de Kleine en Grote Dramaturgie: Pleidooi voor een "Interlocuteur"'. *Etcetera.* 17.68. (1999): 67–69. Print.

———. 'European Dramaturgy in the 21st Century'. *Performance Research.* 14.3. (2009): 7–11. Print.

Venuti, Lawrence. Ed. *Translation Studies Reader.* Florence, KY: Routledge, 1999. Print.

———. *The Translator's Invisibility: A History of Translation.* 2nd Ed. London: Routledge, 2008. Print.

Vincendeau, Ginette. *La Haine.* I.B Tauris, 2005. Print.

Wehrs, Donald R. & Blake, Thomas. Eds. *The Palgrave Handbook of Affect Studies and Textual Criticism.* London: Palgrave Macmillan, 2017. Print.

Welcker, Ellen. 'Only Poems Can Translate Poems: On the Impossibility and Necessity of Translation'. *The Quarterly Conversation.* 2008. Web. Accessed: 23 July 2010. <http://quarterlyconversation.com/only-poems-can-trans-late-poems-on-the-impossibility-and-necessity-of-translation>.

Welsch, Wolfgang. 'Transculturality—The Puzzling Form of Cultures Today'. *Spaces of Culture: City, Nation, World.* Ed. Featherstone, Mike & Scott Lash. London: Sage, 1999. 194–213. Print.

Wildman, Wesley J. 'Theology Without Walls: The Future of Transreligious Theology'. *Open Theology.* 2. (2016): 242–247. Web. Accessed: 28 July 2018. <https://www.degruyter.com/downloadpdf/j/opth.2016.2.issue-1/opth-2016-0019/opth-2016-0019.pdf>.

Wolf, Sara. 'Sidi Larbi Cherkaoui's "Myth": The Choreographer, a Rising Star in EUROPE, Presents a U.S. Premiere at UCLA'. 2008. Web. Accessed: 22 October 2008. <http://www.latimes.com/news/nationworld/world/europe/la-et-myth20-2008oct20,0,885490.story>.

Woolf, Diana. 'Maker of the Month /Kei Ito'. *Ideas in the Making*. 2010. Web. Accessed: 8 August 2018. <http://www.themaking.org.uk/Content/makers/2010/01/kei_ito.html>.

Ziolkowski, Jan. Ed. *Dante and Islam*. New York: Fordham University Press, 2014. Print.

Multimedia Sources

Apocrifu. Choreographed by Sidi Larbi Cherkaoui. 2007. Video Recording of Performance.

Babel^(words). Co-choreographed by Sidi Larbi Cherkaoui and Damien Jalet. 2010. Video Recording of Performance.

'Baby Love'. Performed by The Supremes. Written by Holland-Dozier-Holland. Motown Records. 1964. Song.

Bye Bye Belgium. RTBF. 2006. Online Video. Accessed: 21 December 2012. <http://www.youtube.com/watch?v=O1OcwJPK3Vo>.

Dogville. Written and Directed by Lars von Trier. 2003. Film.

Foi. Choreographed by Sidi Larbi Cherkaoui. 2003. Video Recording of Performance.

Ick seg adieu (Souterliedeken 65). Written by Gherardus Mes. Performed by Camerata Trajectina. Online Video of Song and Translated Lyrics. Accessed: 5 August 2017. <https://www.youtube.com/watch?v=RHeejbPHFQs>.

Is the Qur'an Corrupted? Biblical Characters in the Qur'an. 2006. Web. Accessed: 17 August 2010. <http://www.youtube.com/watch?v=raw-SB7AjMo>.

La Zon-Mai. Created by Sidi Larbi Cherkaoui and Gilles Delmas. Lardux Films. 2007. Web. Accessed: 18 July 2014. <http://www.zon-mai.com/accueil_fr>.

Les Ailes Brisées/Shattered Wings. Created by Gilles Delmas. Lardux Films. 2008. DVD.

Myth. Choreographed by Sidi Larbi Cherkaoui. 2007. Video Recording of Performance.

Pello Joxepe. Traditional Basque Song Performed by Paco Ibañez. 2008. Song. Accessed: 6 June 2008. <http://www.youtube.com/watch?v=ttuRcl1dK1M>.

Rêves de Babel / Dreams of Babel. Created by Sidi Larbi Cherkaoui. Directed by Don Kent. BelAir Media. 2010. DVD.

Rien de Rien. Choreographed by Sidi Larbi Cherkaoui. 2000. Video Recording of Performance.

'Somewhere Over the Rainbow'. Performed by Judy Garland. Written by Harold Arlen & Edgard Yipsel Harburg. Metro-Goldwyn-Mayer. 1939. Song.

Submission. Written by Ayaan Hirsi Ali. Produced by Theo Van Gogh. 2004. Film.

Sutra. Choreographed by Sidi Larbi Cherkaoui. Sadler's Wells. Axiom Films. 2008. DVD.

The Offensive Translator. Written by Catherine Tate. 2006. Web. Accessed: 1 February 2019. <https://www.youtube.com/watch?v=XY66ZJ0TFUI>.

The Wizard of Oz. Directed by Victor Fleming. Metro-Goldwyn-Mayer. 1939. Film.

'We Need a War'. Written and Performed by Fischerspooner. Odyssey. 2005. Song.

'Yerushalayim Shel Zahav'. Written and Performed by Naomi Shemer. 1967. Song.

Zero Degrees. Co-choreographed by Sidi Larbi Cherkaoui and Akram Khan. Sadler's Wells. Axiom Films. 2008. DVD.

Zéro Degré: L'Infini. Created by Gilles Delmas. Lardux Films. 2006. DVD.

Interviews

Cherkaoui, Sidi Larbi. Interview with author 1. Antwerp, May 2004.

———. Interview with author 2. London, June 2004.

———. Interview with author 3. Châteauvallon, July 2004.

———. Interview with author 4. Antwerp, June 2007.

———. Interview with Guy Cools. London, December 2008, part of the body: language series at Sadler's Wells.

Dudley, Joanna. Interview with author. London, June 2004.

Jalet, Damien. Interview with author. London, June 2004.

Leboutte, Christine. Interview with author. London, June 2004.

Neyskens, Laura. Interview with author. London, June 2004.

Ómarsdóttir, Erna. Interview with author. London, June 2004.

Seabra, Helder. Interview with author. Brussels, March 2010.

Snellings, Dirk. Telephone interview with author. June 2004.

Van Outryve, Jan. Interview with author. London, June 2004.

Index